Facilitating Self Care
Practices in the Elderly

Facilitating Self Care Practices in the Elderly

Barbara J. Horn, RN, PhD
Editor

Elderly Home Care Project
Principal Investigator: Barbara J. Horn, RN, PhD
Funded by Fred Meyer Charitable Trust
Sponsoring Agency: University of Washington
Department of Community Health Care Systems
Seattle, WA 98195

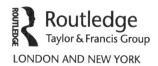

Routledge
Taylor & Francis Group

LONDON AND NEW YORK

Facilitating Self Care Practices in the Elderly has also been published as *Home Health Care Services Quarterly*, Volume 11, Numbers 1/2 1990.

First published 1990 by The Haworth Press, Inc.

Published 2018 by Routledge
2 Park Square, Milton Park, Abingdon, Oxon, OX14 4RN
52 Vanderbilt Avenue, New York, NY 10017

First issued in paperback 2018

Routledge is an imprint of the Taylor & Francis Group, an informa business

Library of Congress Cataloging-in-Publication Data

Facilitating self-care practices in the elderly / Barbara J. Horn, editor.
    p. cm.
    "Has also been published as Home health care services quarterly, volume 11, numbers 1/2, 1990" – T.p. verso.
    Includes bibliographical references.
    ISBN 1-56024-013-X
    1. Aged – Home care. I. Horn, Barbara J.
RA564.8.F33   1990
649.8 – dc20   90-4244
                                                 CIP

ISBN 13: 978-1-138-96945-2 (pbk)
ISBN 13: 978-1-56024-013-6 (hbk)

Facilitating Self Care Practices in the Elderly

CONTENTS

ABOUT THE EDITOR

Barbara J. Horn, RN, PhD, is Professor in the Community Health Care Systems Department in the School of Nursing at the University of Washington in Seattle, Washington. Dr. Horn is also the program coordinator for the Rural Hospital Initiative, a program through The Northwest Geriatric Education Center, also at the University of Washington, Seattle. As an educator and researcher, she has taught and conducted studies in the reorganization of nursing services; the evaluation of the impact of change on cost, quality of care, and nurse satisfaction; and the development and testing of criterion measures to assess quality in all care settings. As an informal care giver for many years, Dr. Horn has developed insight into the issues pertinent to providing quality care, particularly in the areas of community-based care and home health care for older adults.

Preface

The purpose and goal of home care as an important segment in
the continuum of health care delivery has remained virtually un-
changed since its modern inception in the mid-1960s—i.e., to assist
persons in their recovery from, or adaptation to, illness in their own
setting. What has changed dramatically is the social, technological,
and regulatory environment in which these services are provide today. Persons are living longer, and with age comes an increase in
the number and kinds of chronic illnesses with which they must
live. Additionally, many elders experience increasing social isolation as a result of outliving their spouses and friendship networks.
Families, the traditional care providers of their members, are in-
creasingly unavailable to assume these responsibilities because of
geographic distance, the conflicting demands of work and/or their
primary family needs. Technological advances, ranging from the
increase of medical specialists to sophisticated drug therapies and
the application of high-technology treatments, have increased the
complexity of care management. Further, economic and regulatory
constraints have forced earlier hospital discharges of patients with a
wide range of medical and social needs. All of these factors have
increased the pressures on home care providers to manage increas-
ingly complex care needs for a population whose ability and readiness to learn are compromised by age, disability, and psychosocial
factors. Home care clinical providers are confronted with the need
to meet conflicting demands of patients and families, regulators,
payors, and their own professional ethics and values of what constitutes quality care. It is not difficult for home care clinical providers,
especially nurses experiencing diverse expectations, to compromise
the essence of their primary role as teacher and advocate to their
clients.

Through their clinical knowledge, understanding of the health
care industry, research expertise, and vision of the potentials for

ix

home health care, the authors have put forth a series of articles addressing primary practice issues relevant in today's complex climate. Not only do they identify the most pressing issues, but they offer specific intervention strategies to address these problems. The articles address the following clinical problems in home care: medication management, tailoring teaching to the elderly, and family coping.

Although each article is unique in its content, each has a similar format which includes theoretical frameworks for examining the problem, practical clinical assessment tools to assist clinicians to specifically define the problem to be addressed, clinical intervention strategies, and planning and policy applications at the organization level. The underlying theme of each article focuses on the unique needs of the elderly based on sensory, cognitive, functional, and psychosocial changes which occur with aging. Intervention strategies are tailored to those characteristics.

This series of articles is directed to, and written for, providers practicing in the home. The content will help increase the provider's knowledge and understanding of the challenges associated with aging and methods of tailoring their interventions to more effectively address those needs. These articles are crucial reading for nurses and other providers who wish to realize an increased sense of personal and professional achievement and satisfaction in assisting their home care clients to better manage their health care needs at home.

Patty Mulher, RN, MN
Director of Patient Services
Visiting Nurse Services
Seattle, WA

Chapter I

Introduction

Barbara J. Horn, RN, PhD

Principal Author

Formal home health care services have been provided for clients and families since the late 19th century in this country. Although elderly persons have been a major group to receive such services, it was not until 1966 that government policy focused on facilitating home care of elderly persons. In 1966, home health care agencies became eligible for Medicare funds. In 1981, the Home Care Waiver allowed Medicare reimbursement for home health care which did not exceed the cost of institutional care.

During the period from 1966 to 1981, Medicare costs for health care of elderly persons more than doubled. In an attempt to control costs, prospective payment systems were instituted for institutional care. Hospitals and medical centers were strongly encouraged to limit the length of hospitalizations according to DRG classifications. As a result of the cost containment policies, elders have been leaving hospitals in an earlier stage of recuperation and have an increased need for formal home care. In addition, the care needs have become more complex; the use of sophisticated high tech equipment such as intravenous systems has become much more common and has contributed to problems of caregivers in the home. Not only do clients and caregivers need to be taught how to provide

This paper is a portion of the material developed by the project staff of the Elderly Home Care Project, Principal Investigator, Barbara J. Horn. Funded by Fred Meyer Charitable Trust. Sponsoring agency: University of Washington, Department of Community Health Care Systems, Seattle, WA 98195.

care in the home, but the interventions and equipment used in the hospital setting usually require modification for use in the home by the elderly.

The work presented in this book is a portion of the material developed by project staff of the three year, Elderly Homecare Project funded by Fred Meyer Charitable Trust (1986-1989).* Major goals of the project were: (1) to identify the impact of early hospital discharge on the provision of home health care by identifying the types of clinical problems home health care providers encountered in providing services to acutely ill, homebound elders, and (2) to develop approaches for managing critical clinical problems identified by home health care agencies. In this chapter, the project design and the findings will be presented. In the ensuing three chapters (II, III, & IV) a review of the "state-of-the-art" and assessment guides for three of the most critical clinical problems will be presented.

DESIGN

The project design was to obtain from home care providers the nine most critical clinical problems facing them as they provided care to elders recently discharged from the hospital setting. Following the generation of the nine problems (master problem list), the literature was reviewed and experts were consulted to determine the current knowledge base. Papers (state-of-the-art) were written for the three most critical problems. Care protocols and education materials were to accompany the papers.

Delphi Process

To identify the clinical problems, 178 Medicare certified home health agencies in Alaska, Idaho, Montana, Oregon, and Washington were asked to participate in the project. A modified Delphi process was used to collect the data. The Delphi process is a set of procedures for formulating a group judgment about a particular subject area. Three rounds of questionnaires were used.

---

*Elderly Homecare Project. Barbara J. Horn, PhD, Principal Investigator. Funded by Fred Meyer Charitable Trust (1986-1989). Grant Number 85070332.

Round I

The first questionnaire used open-ended questions. An agency contact person was asked to identify clinical problems (physiological, psychosocial, or technological) that providers of their home care agency were experiencing in relation to early hospital discharge of the elderly client. The problems identified by the agencies were categorized through a process of content analysis. Three revisions of the categories were necessary in order to achieve a category system that could accommodate the data. Two coders then used the category system to classify each problem documented in the responses. Agreement between the two coders was achieved through consensus. One limitation of the data is that clients and care givers were not asked for their perceptions of their needs. The five major categories which evolved from the data were:

1. Technologically sophisticated, complex or time-intensive nursing problem.
2. Problems involving psychosocial and client/family issues.
3. Problems related to client/family teaching.
4. Problems related to the health care delivery system.
5. Problems of miscellaneous nature.

The response rate for round I was 60% (118 out of 178 agencies responded).

Round II

The second round questionnaire was closed-ended. The top ranking 30 clinical problems within the first three categories, namely: (1) technologically sophisticated, complex, time-intensive nursing problems; (2) psychosocial problems; and (3) teaching problems, were submitted to the agencies. Agencies were instructed to indicate if each of the 30 problems listed was a current problem for their agency. If the agency indicated that it was a problem, the agency was instructed to rate (using a five-point rating scale) three dimensions. These dimensions were: (1) complexity of the problem, (2) degree of technology required, and (3) frequency of problem occurrence. The response rate for round II was 84% (99 out of 118 agencies responded).

Round III

The third questionnaire was developed from the responses from round II and contained the 15 highest ranked clinical problems. The 15 problems were selected as follows: the problem had to be mentioned by at least 50% of the agencies responding to Round II. Agencies were again asked to indicate if the problem was currently a problem for their agency and if it was a problem, to rate the problems for the three dimensions — complexity, technology, and frequency. On Round III, the agencies were given information on how their agency and other agencies had rated the problem on the second round. Thus, agencies had information about other agencies' views in relation to the problem. The response rate for Round III was 89% (88 out of 99 agencies responded).

Nine problems were selected from responses of the agencies to Round III. Criteria used for the selection for these problems were:

1. That the problem was rated at "3" or above on the 5 point rating scale for two of the three dimensions — complexity, technology, and frequency.
2. That the problem ranked among the top ten of the fifteen problems.

Utilizing the modified Delphi process we gained consensus from experts about their perception of the most pressing clinical problems in providing home care to elders.

FINDINGS

Sample Characteristics

The sample characteristics are based on 118 responses of Round I. The response rate was representative of all five states in the region. The sample agencies were providing care to the elderly as evidenced by the data which indicated that 84% of the clients served were 65 years of age or older.

The type of agency in the sample represented was that 60% were community based of which 30% were for profit, and 40% were hospital based of which 88% were not for profit. Forty-nine percent were rural while 51% were urban.

An analysis of the representativeness of the sample in relation to major demographic variables was conducted using cross tabulation and the Chi-Square statistic as well as the Kruskal-Wallis One-Way ANOVA and the Mann-Whitney U Test for group differences. The use of these tests over parametric counterparts was mandated by failure to meet the assumptions of normality and heterogeneous of variances. Major findings were generally consistent across all three rounds.

Statistical testing revealed no significant differences across states in regard to community based, hospital based or for profit or not for profit agencies. There were significant differences in the number of rural versus urban agencies by state, with proportionately more rural agencies than expected by chance in Idaho, Montana, and Oregon and proportionately more urban agencies than expected by chance in Washington. Significant differences were found in the number of for profit/not for profit agencies by community versus hospital based. More for profit agencies were community based while more not-for-profit were hospital based.

Master Problem List

At the completion of the third round of questionnaires the following nine clinical problems emerged as the most critical:

1. Teaching elders and families medication regimens
2. Nursing management of elder coping problems
3. Nursing management of family coping problems
4. Nursing management of intravenous therapies
5. Teaching elder/family management of intravenous therapies
6. Nursing management of symptoms for clients with cancer
7. Nursing management of wounds
8. Teaching elders/family care of wounds
9. Teaching elders/family management of diabetes

DISCUSSION

In the following three chapters, three of the top problems will be discussed.** Medication self-administration will be discussed in Chapter II. Medication regimens constitute a major treatment modality for most patients served by home care agencies. While medication regimens may be beneficial for treating disease processes, the problem for the patient, family, and health providers associated with maintaining an adequate medication program are complex and varied. Two major concerns were expressed by the sample regarding medication regimens. These concerns were: (1) medication non-compliance of the client and/or family members who were not supportive to the client in adhering to the medication regimen, and (2) the health providers' lack of knowledge of intervention strategies and/or lack of education materials for assisting patients and families with medication management. The content includes a synthesis of the literature related to medication-taking behavior of the elders and factors related to medication compliance. An assessment guide is presented followed by suggested intervention strategies and sources for education materials.

Because teaching was a component of three out of the nine major problems listed, the project team decided that a special state-of-the-art paper was needed on teaching the elderly. Therefore, Chapter III was written to assist home care providers in developing better and more effective teaching strategies. The literature was reviewed on special teaching techniques and adaptations for elderly in general and for elders with sensory, mobility or cognitive difficulties. Important guidelines for teaching are summarized. The appendix of Chapter III provides sample teaching plans, examples of how to assess and develop educational materials for reading level and lists teaching resources for clinicians and clients.

Family coping when providing care to older members is the focus of Chapter IV. Management of family coping problems when pro-

---

**Five additional papers will be published in future issues of *Home Health Care Services Quarterly*. The papers will address problems related to assisting elders to care for wounds, cancer symptom management, home intravenous therapy, and elderly clients coping with illness.

viding care to elderly members was identified as a major problem for home care staff. Staff identified families as being stressed, fearful, apprehensive, anxious, burned out, fatigued, and feeling overwhelmed. These feelings were attributed to: (1) the families' lack of understanding or knowledge of needed care and (2) the lack of community or family resources that could help family members cope or have time away from caregiving. Therefore, Chapter IV focuses on the magnitude and significance of family caregiving problems and theoretical frameworks that provide explanations of family coping problems. An assessment guide was developed to assist the home care staff in working with families. The methods and results of developing the assessment guide for use by home care agency staff also are discussed in Chapter IV.

THE IMPORTANCE OF COLLABORATIVE EFFORT

Although these papers were authored by faculty in an academic setting, they could not have been developed and written without the combined knowledge of researchers, clinicians and educators in home health care. Bringing these three areas of expertise together was essential to the process of applying current theory and research findings to the important problems of home health care for the elderly.

An understanding of the research process was required for examining current literature for relevant conceptual frameworks, for deciding on the research design for obtaining consensus from home care agencies, for developing and testing the medication and family caregiver assessment guides, and for integrating teaching and learning concepts for older populations. The experience of clinicians who dealt with the day to day problems that the elderly must confront was required for deciding which problems were most important to address, for developing assessments that were practical for clinicians to use, and for testing and evaluating those assessments in clinical settings. The educational environment contained the necessary link between research and practice through its provision of faculty time for initiating and generating financial support for investigating the problems, bringing experts together to work on the problems, and for disseminating the information about the results of the project.

In summary, the papers that follow illustrate how a regional approach and collaborative efforts can be combined to identify problems and bring current information to clinical agencies and their staff. With the growing proportion of elderly in the population and the complexity of the problems that need solutions, no single expert or field of inquiry can hope to find workable answers in time to meet the changing needs.

Chapter II

Medication Regimens
and the Home Care Client:
A Challenge for Health Care Providers

Betty L. Pesznecker, MN
Carol Patsdaughter, PhD
Kimberly A. Moody, MS
Marilynn Albert, MS

Principal Authors

Jana R. Ostrom, RPh, MS

Consultant

Kathleen O'Connor, MA

Editor

SUMMARY. This paper synthesizes literature related to medication-taking behaviors of the elderly population and examines factors
related to medication compliance problems. A review and critique
of the literature focused on interventions and strategies for improving medication compliance is also presented. This analysis provides
direction for developing assessment guides, intervention strategies,
and educational materials which may be helpful for health providers
in assisting patients and families to manage medication regimens.
The paper also includes a comprehensive medication assessment

---

This paper is a portion of the material developed by the project staff of the
Elderly Home Care Project, Principal Investigator, Barbara J. Horn. Funded by
Fred Meyer Charitable Trust. Sponsoring agency: University of Washington, De-
partment of Community Health Care Systems, Seattle, WA 98195.

9

guide and a resource list of educational materials for family caregivers and health providers. The last section of the paper describes the clinical testing study of the medication assessment guide.

Medication regimens constitute a major treatment modality for most patients served by home care agencies. While medication regimens may be beneficial for treating disease processes, the problems for the patient, family and health provider associated with maintaining an adequate medication program are complex and varied.

The Delphi survey of Medicare-certified home care agencies in the Northwest Region, as described in Chapter I, indicated that medication problems were ranked highest of all clinical problems in relation to earlier discharge of elderly patients from hospitals. Two major concerns regarding medication regimens were expressed: (a) medication non-compliance of the patient and/or family members who were not supportive to the patient in adhering to the medication regimen, and (b) the health providers' lack of knowledge of intervention strategies and/or lack of educational materials for assisting patients and families with medication management.

In this chapter, the literature related to medication-taking behavior of the elderly population and factors related to medication compliance problems are synthesized. A review and critique of the literature focused on interventions and strategies for improving medication compliance is also presented. This analysis provided direction for the development of the Comprehensive Medication Assessment Guide (see Attachment A). The development and testing of the guide is reported in the last section of the chapter.

USE OF MEDICATIONS AND PREVALENCE OF MEDICATION PROBLEMS IN OLDER PEOPLE

Those over 65 years of age constitute 11 percent of the United States population, yet 25 to 30 percent of health care expenditures are for this age group (Kovar, 1977). It has been estimated that the elderly in developed countries also consume 25 to 30 percent of total expenditures for drugs and drug products (Vestal, 1982). Between 1978 and 1982, the number of prescribed medications for the total population in England increased by 2.6 percent, while those for the elderly increased by 3.9 percent (DHSS, 1978 & 1982). In the United States, 75.2 percent of non-institutionalized persons over 65 had at least one medication prescribed and the mean number of prescription medications acquired yearly by persons over 65 was 10.7 (Kasper, 1982).

A British study of 120 community-based elderly clients demonstrated that 12.5 percent took no medications within the 24 hour period surveyed, while 74.1 percent took 1 to 3 medications and 13.3 percent took four or more medications. The average intake was two medications per patient (Wade & Finlayson, 1983). Other studies substantiate these findings. Kendrick and Bayne (1982) studied 40 patients in a home care program and reported an average intake of 3.8 prescription medications and 1.2 non-prescription drugs. In a survey of 559 subjects over the age of 65 living in New Zealand, respondents between the age of 65 and 79 took 1.5 medications; those over the age of 80 took 2.1 mediations, mostly diuretics, digoxin and psychotropic medications (Campbell, McCosh, & Reinken, 1983). However, Ostrom, Hammarlund, Christensen, Plein, and Kethley (1985) surveyed 183 independently living elderly residents of two federally subsidized, urban high-rise apartment buildings in the United States and reported an average of 3.1 prescription medications and 2.6 non-prescription drugs taken.

Non-prescription drugs tend to be heavily used by persons over 65. Estimates suggest that up to 75 percent of individuals 65 and over use non-prescription medications. Some individuals may routinely use more than 10 of these drugs (Simonson, 1984). In addition, the elderly use over-the-counter drugs at a rate that may be seven times greater than that of younger adults. Eight percent of older non-prescription medication users also use alcohol, prescribed medications, or both (Kofoed, 1985).

With increasing age, elderly persons tend to take more prescription medications. Furthermore, the consensus of a number of descriptive studies is that elderly people have a variety of problems related to the management of their drug regimens. One study, a structured interview of 114 randomly selected outpatients over 65 years of age, revealed that 20 percent of the respondents reported that they forgot to take their medication or took too little or too much (Klein, German, Levine, Feroli, & Ardery, 1984). Data from a structured interview study of 50 patients over 65 years of age, indicated that 25 percent of the medications were not being taken as labeled (Lundin, 1978). A study of 138 subjects taking prescription medications regularly also indicated high use. Fifty-one percent were taking medication in dosages other than those which appeared on the prescription container (Ostrom, Hammarlund, Christensen, Plein, & Kethley, 1985). Other problems reported in this study were: (a) overuse and underuse of medication, (b) inability to read label or open childproof container, (c) lack of knowledge about the purpose of the medication, (d) poor storage of medications, (e) outdated prescriptions, and (f) sharing medications with others. These findings have also been cited all as specifically associated with medication management in elderly persons in other studies (Lamy, 1984; Smith & Sharpe, 1984; Fletcher, Fletcher, Thomas, & Hamann, 1979; Squire, Goldman, Kupersmith, Stern, Fuster, & Schweitzer, 1984; Parkin, Henney, Quirk & Crooks, 1976).

Improper management of the medication regimen may exacerbate the disease process, or precipitate a drug reaction. Frisk, Cooper, and Campbell (1977) studied 392 patients admitted to two community hospitals. One out of five patients had a drug-related problem which probably precipitated the hospital admission. The problems included adverse response to prescribed therapy, misuse of medication or non-compliance, effect of diet on therapy, patient treatment by more than one provider, and therapeutic ineffectiveness, or inappropriateness of prescribed therapy. In a similar study, McKenney and Harrison (1976) examined the association between hospital admissions and drug-related problems of 216 patients. Fifty-nine patients were found to have a drug-related problem. Adverse drug reactions and non-compliance appeared to be the principal factors in hospital admission.

ADVERSE DRUG REACTIONS IN THE ELDERLY

The above findings indicate an increasing incidence of adverse drug reactions in the elderly. These findings are alarming because the elderly tend to be more susceptible to adverse drug reactions than younger persons. Persons 60 to 70 years of age are twice as likely to have adverse drug reactions than the younger population.

The risk is tripled for persons over 80 years of age as compared to people under 50 (Wade & Bowling, 1986). While medication usage rate is a factor, increased risk can be attributed to a number of other factors, including physiological changes, drug interactions, nutritional status and problems with compliance. (See Table 1.)

Age-related drug absorption alteration may take a variety of forms. Gastric mobility tends to slow with age, prolonging transit time for drugs absorbed in the bowel. Gastric pH increases with age thereby potentially altering the solubility of some drugs. Splanchnic blood flow is decreased, which could delay or decrease absorption. Active and passive transport of some materials in the gastro-intestinal tract is slowed, so that transfer of some chemically-related drugs may also be slowed. Although all of these changes could change drug metabolism, there are few studies that suggest such alterations do, in fact, occur (Ouslander, 1981; Simonson, 1984; Vestal, 1982).

Drugs also tend to be distributed differently in the elderly due to changes in body size and composition and serum protein composition. In general, older people are smaller than younger people because of age-related decreases in stature and the tendency of succeeding generations to be larger than those that preceded them. Practitioners, therefore, should proceed cautiously in prescribing drug doses to an older population since most dosage standards have been developed for young adults (Simonson, 1984; Ouslander, 1981).

Gradual significant changes in body composition also occur with aging. There is an increase in percentage of body fat, and a corresponding decrease in body water. These changes may significantly alter the distribution of specific drugs in an older client (Simonson, 1984; Ouslander, 1981).

In elderly persons, there is a decreased amount of albumin in the bloodstream, probably due to the decreased production of albumin by the liver. There is some evidence that decreased serum albumin alters the way some drugs (especially those that are protein-bound) are carried in the bloodstream and also changes the amount of a drug required to have a therapeutic effect in an older patient (Simonson, 1984; Ouslander, 1981).

In order to be utilized and excreted, many drugs must be metabo-

TABLE 1

Reasons for Increased Rate of Adverse Medication Reactions among the Elderly

Absorption

Gastric mobility ↓

Gastric pH ↑

Splanchnic blood flow ↓

Slowed transport out ↓
of intestine

Distribution

Smaller stature ↓

% body fat ↑

% body water ↓

serum albumen ↓

Metabolism

Hepatic function ↓

Renal clearance 50% ↓

Interaction with Medication

Nutrition effect on
medication absorption

Nutrition effect on
medication metabolism

Alteration of food
metabolism by medications

Medication Interaction

risk due to larger average
# of medications used

risk due to common usage of
interaction prone medications

Noncompliance

Intentional

Nonintentional

lized in the liver. There may be a decrease in liver function with age, which may change the rate at which a drug is processed. The change is thought to be a consequence of a decrease in hepatic blood flow, hepatic mass and enzyme activity. Some drugs that require metabolism in the liver before excretion have been found to have higher concentrations in the elderly since the liver is not processing them efficiently (Simonson, 1984).

Decrease in renal function is a well recognized correlate of aging. It is accompanied by a 50 percent decrease in clearance rate of most medications from the blood stream leading to a higher serum concentration of drugs. Decreased renal function is mostly caused by a decrease in renal circulation (Simonson, 1984, Ouslander, 1981).

As pointed out by Vestal (1984), elderly persons not only have normal age related changes which affect their absorption, distribution and elimination of drugs, but they also may have one or more chronic illnesses. Chronic disease processes may further compromise organ function, which only exacerbates the problems of drug absorption, distribution, and elimination, thus putting the elderly person at even further risk for adverse drug reactions (Vestal, 1984).

As the number of drugs a client takes increases, so does his or her risk for an adverse drug interaction. Since the elderly, as a group, tend to take more medication than the general population, they are more prone to interactions. Moreover, certain classes of drugs (such as digoxin, diuretics, and central nervous system depressants) which are frequently involved in interactions, are very commonly prescribed in the elderly, further increasing the risk of interaction (Wade & Finlayson, 1983).

Diet also has a significant impact on drug absorption. Nutrients typically interact with drugs in three ways. First, the presence or absence of nutrients in the gastrointestinal tract can significantly affect the absorption of many drugs. Some drugs are bound in the intestine by certain substances, some are better absorbed on an empty stomach, and some are better absorbed or tolerated when taken with food. Second, drug metabolism or excretion can be changed by changing the food intake of an individual. For example, decreasing the salt content of the diet changes the excretion of lithium which can result in toxic levels of this drug remaining in the blood. Finally, drugs can alter food metabolism, thereby causing nutritional deficiencies (Lamy, 1982; Roe, 1986).

Improper self-administration of medications also contributes to adverse drug reaction. Taking too much or too little of a medication, or administering it at the wrong time, or not at all, may contribute to drug reactions and other related problems. The special circumstances of the elderly in relation to medication indicates the necessity for assistance in developing and maintaining a medication regimen. Home care nurses need to be especially attuned to the problems of adverse drug reaction and communicate concerns to the physician who prescribed the medication.

COMPLIANCE

The home care nurse is in a key role to determine possible non-compliance associated with the medication regimen. Medication non-compliance, however, is a multifaceted, complex phenomenon which requires careful and thorough assessment and individualized treatment strategies based on that assessment. In order to assist in assessment and treatment strategies effectively, the remainder of this paper focuses on developing an operational definition of medication non-compliance in the elderly, factors associated with it, and strategies to improve compliance.

Operational Definition of Compliance

Compliance is a term surrounded with controversy. Haynes, Taylor, and Sackett (1979) defined compliance as the extent to which a person's behavior conforms or does not conform to the advice of the health care provider. To some researchers, compliance has been interpreted as placing the entire responsibility for conforming or nonconforming on the individual (Morisky, Green, & Levine, 1986). Although this "victim blaming" may exist in some situations, the term "non-compliance," as used in this paper, does not have that connotation.

Some authors used the word "adherence" in place of the word "compliance" in order to avoid the controversy (Morisky, Green & Levine, 1986; Blackwell, 1976). These authors have expressed concern that there are also coercive connotations to the word "compliance" and that the term "adherence" seems more neutral.

"Compliance" is used in this paper since it is the most widely used of the two terminologies in the literature. Its use is intended to indicate the extent to which a patient's behavior conforms to the prescribed regimen. It is used in a descriptive manner and no value judgement is implied.

The remainder of this section will explore the concept of compliance as follows: (a) types of compliance problems, (b) methods of measuring compliance, and (c) ethical issues regarding compliance.

Types of Compliance Problems

Christensen (1978) reported that compliance problems are categorized in many different ways. These differences pose particular problems when attempting to generalize findings. Some investigators have included only errors of omission, which refer to omitting a prescribed dose of a drug. Others have included errors of commission, which refer to taking drugs in addition to those prescribed by the physician, or taking drugs incorrectly. Errors of commission include errors of dosage and timing. Understanding the differences between these types of errors is important in identifying the focus on intervention.

Errors of omission occur when a patient misses one or more scheduled medications. These errors can happen for a variety of reasons. There may be a problem in the physician/patient communication resulting in misunderstanding. For example, the medication order said "take with meals" and the patient has only two meals a day which means the patient took the medication twice a day instead of three times a day. Errors of omission can occur because the patient could not remove the childproof cap from the container or because the patient could not read the fine print on the label. Increasing forgetfulness, lack of understanding about the treatment, suspicions and mistrust of drugs or of those administering them, adverse reactions, or expense can all contribute towards these errors (Wade & Bowling, 1986). There are obviously a multitude of possible reasons for errors of omission, which create quite a challenge to the nurse assessing the situation.

Errors of commission occur when a patient takes too much or too little of a medication or takes additional drugs which confound the intended effect of the prescribed medication. Thus, errors of commission include dosage errors such as taking the wrong amount of the drug and timing errors such as taking the drug at the wrong time. In addition, medications may be taken that are outdated. Since elderly are known to sometimes share medications with friends or to use different providers who are unaware of other prescriptions the patient may be taking, there is a need to assess what different over-the-counter drugs they may be taking as well as what combinations of drugs they may be using. Drug overuse is often the outcome of a patient believing "more must be even better" or of a physician/patient miscommunication. Furthermore, elderly clients are particularly at risk for errors of omission and commission because of the frequency of changes in their multiple medication regimens. Additionally, elderly clients who have been discharged from institutional settings may have entirely new medication regimens or have their old regimens drastically changed. Thus, nurses need to use skillful assessment techniques to determine the underlying cause for medication errors and try to identify which type of combinations of errors are occurring.

Cooper, Love and Raffoul (1982) stressed the importance of differentiating between nonintentional versus intentional non-compliance. They defined intentional non-compliance as underuse or overuse that was at a "conscious level and deliberate." Unintentional non-compliance was defined as non-compliance for which there was no conscious intent (p. 330).

There is a tendency among health care workers to assume that if patients want to become healthier, they logically desire to follow the medication regimen in pursuit of this goal. This assumption has been shown not to be the case for many patients. For one reason or another, patients often decide to stop taking their medications. Sometimes the side effects are so negative that they outweigh the positive therapeutic impact. In other cases, the patient does not really believe in the medical regimen. Other reasons for intentionally not taking medications are related to the expense of the medication or difficulty in getting prescriptions refilled.

Cooper, Love, and Raffoul (1982) studied non-compliant behavior by older persons and found a large proportion (73%) of non-compliance was intentional. In the reported list of reasons for non-compliance, the largest category was the client's perception that the drug was not needed in the dosage required. These researchers pointed out that traditional methods aimed at reducing the incidence of forgetting to take medicines would not seem helpful in cases of intentional non-compliance.

There may be many reasons why clients decide not to comply, but they are reluctant to talk about these realities to nurses and physicians whose jobs are seen to promote compliance. Cooper, Love and Raffoul (1982) suggested the possibility that intentional non-compliance in the elderly may be an effective adaptation when — due to normal aging variations in physiological absorption, distribution, and excretion of the drug — there may be need for a less frequent dosage schedule. Further investigation regarding the relationship between non-compliance and health behavior is warranted. These situations also require special skills at assessing compliance patterns with an understanding of the multiplicity of interacting variables.

Methods of Assessing Compliance Problems

There are several methods of assessing compliance problems. The methods are complex and involve different areas of concern. One area of concern is identifying the extent to which the client complies with the prescribed regimen. Another area of concern is assessing the nature of factors which facilitate and inhibit compliance. The following section briefly summarizes some methods for measuring compliance with medication-taking and analyzes the clinical implications associated with them.

Methods of assessing non-compliance can be grouped into two categories: direct and indirect methods. Direct methods are those by which the medication can be detected in the client (Evans & Spelman, 1983). Indirect methods include some form of assessment, either by the client or by someone else, as to whether the client is likely to have taken the medication (Evans & Spelman, 1983).

Direct Methods

Direct methods include blood level monitoring and analysis of excretions. The concentration of a drug or its metabolites in the blood will often give some indication of the actual dose being taken by the client. When it is too difficult to identify a substance in the blood, a compound that can be more easily identified is added to the therapeutic agent and acts as a marker. Measurements of excretion take various forms. It is possible to identify certain drugs which are excreted in the urine or stools or even breath. The phenothiazides and tricyclic antidepressants are examples of drugs which can be detected in the urine. Some drugs can be identified in the urine by their excreted metabolites.

In some cases, marker compounds have been used by attaching them to the therapeutic agents enabling the urinary excretion of the drug to be measured. An attempt has been made to mark the stools of psychiatric clients by giving the client an opaque barium sulphate tracer detectable by x-rays in the feces (Evans & Spelman, 1983). A breath test can identify drugs or drug metabolites in the expired air of clients taking disulfiram. Blood tests, urine tests, stool markers, and breath tests all provide objective and fairly reliable evidence of compliance. However, they are costly and inconvenient, making these tests impractical for most clinical uses (Christensen, 1978).

Indirect Methods

Indirect methods of compliance assessment include: (a) pill counts, (b) outcome criteria based on therapeutic expectations, (c) the presence of expected side effects, and (d) interview of client or relatives (Evans & Spelman, 1983).

Pill counts involve asking the client to return a medication container at regular intervals. The medication not used is counted and provides a basis for an assessment of compliance. One technique is to give the client more medication than required for the period under study and to count the tablets left in the bottle when returned (Evans & Spelman, 1983).

Therapeutic outcomes from drug treatment can be used as a basis for assessing compliance. For example, blood pressure changes are often used as criteria of compliance with antihypertensive medication treatment. With certain drugs, side effects occur consistently when the client is on a therapeutic dosage; assessment of these side effects may give an indication of the extent of compliance (Evans & Spelman, 1983). All these methods have limitations. Pill counts do not always represent what is expected. There may be missing pills from accidental dropping or because clients may dispose of medications they have not taken to give the impression that they have been complying. Pill counts reveal nothing about whether or not drugs were taken at the correct times or in the correct amounts. Expected outcomes of therapy and expected side effects can be unreliable due to the many variables which influence such signs. For example, hypertension is influenced by many factors such as stress management, dietary alterations, and exercise. Outcomes may not be indicative of any one factor.

Interviewing has been shown to be the most promising method of assessing compliance because it is relatively easy to perform and fairly reliable as a measure. According to Haynes, Sackett, and Taylor (1980), about one-half of non-compliant clients will admit that they are not taking at least some of their medications. These authors report that clients who admit their non-compliance on direct questioning are the most responsive to intervention techniques. A matter-of-fact, non-judgmental, non-threatening approach is recommended in questioning to allow the client to "save face." It is emphasized that even clients who admit to non-compliance tend to overestimate their actual compliance. Some suggested interview questions include the following: "Many people find it difficult to take medicines. Do you ever miss or forget to take your pills?" If the client answers in the affirmative, probe for specifics. "How frequently does this happen?" "What are the reasons for missing medications?" (Haynes, Sackett, & Taylor, 1980).

Mathews and Hingson (1977) suggested asking questions aimed at identifying potential non-complying clients and related variables which can direct interventions. These questions address: (a) anxiety about the illness, (b) perceptions of the seriousness of the illness, (c) perceptions of the efficacy of the regimen, and (d) potential barrier the client may anticipate in following the medication regimen.

Morisky, Green, and Levine (1986) developed and tested a four item questionnaire which shows promise as a valid and useful measure of compliance. Items in their self-report scale address patterns of medication-taking behavior (forgetting to take medications and prematurely stopping to take the medication) and permit the health care provider to reinforce positive compliance behaviors.

Ebert (1980), outlined a guide for obtaining a medication history. The history includes questions that elicit information about: (a) medications currently being taken; (b) medications taken during the past year; (c) accuracy of medication self-administration; (d) problems related to medication self-administration, including forgetting, finances, storage, etc.; (e) adverse reactions; and (f) use of over-the-counter medicines. The guide may be useful to gather data as a basis for determining the specific self-administration problems that elder home care clients may be experiencing.

Client interviews seem to be the most useful of the various methods of assessing compliance, but interviews may be more reliable when used in combination with other methods. There is a need for more study and testing in this area.

ETHICAL ISSUES RELATED TO COMPLIANCE

Whether clients should always comply with their medication prescriptions is an issue that currently is receiving attention in research literature (King & Peck, 1981). Gerber and Nehemkis (1986) discussed some of the very complex dilemmas surrounding compliance. According to these authors, clients may be justified in defaulting on a number of grounds, especially invalid diagnosis and inappropriate prescriptions. Clients are not and should not be passive unquestioning recipients of medical instruction (King & Peck, 1981). Haynes, Sackett, and Taylor (1980) responded to these ethical concerns by stating their conceptions of the required preconditions for the application of compliance-enhancing strategies: (a) correct diagnosis of the disease, (b) prescription of effective therapy, (c) an informed client willing to participate in attempts to promote compliance.

Home care nurses who encounter clients with possible ineffective therapy or questionable diagnosis of disease should advocate for clients by: (a) calling the physician to discuss client concerns, or (b) encouraging clients to call the physician to discuss their concerns. Home care nurses also play a key role in providing information to home care clients about disease processes and treatment regimens. Such information may promote client participation in compliance-enhancing strategies.

Gerber and Nehemkis (1986) raised an important issue about the value differences which have consistently been ignored in health care provider's goals for clients who, over long periods of time, resist compliance with the prescribed regimen but continue to seek help with their health problems. This issue concerns the expectations health care providers have for compliance behaviors, which in the face of non-compliant behavior, results in attitudes of anger, frustration, and resentment. It is suggested that most clients with long term chronic illnesses have different perspectives about the self-denial and future-emphasis values necessary for them to comply with their medical regimens. These non-compliers are often labeled as problem clients without examination of the differences between staff expectations and client goals (Gerber & Nehemkis, 1986).

FACTORS CONTRIBUTING TO NON-COMPLIANCE WITH MEDICATION-TAKING

Non-compliance with medication taking is widespread. Although problems of non-compliance have received considerable attention in the health literature, these problems remain poorly understood. Factors affecting whether clients take their medications or not are multiple and complex. The research findings in this area are often contradictory and ambiguous, probably as a result of conceptual and methodological problems. A review of the research, however, provides some insight into persistent factors which seem to be related to non-compliance behavior.

Factors contributing to non-compliance can be organized into three major categories: (a) Client Characteristic Focused, (b) Provider/Treatment Focused and (c) Environmental/Situational Focused. (See Table 2, Summary of Factors Related to Medication Non-Compliance.) These categories provide a framework within

TABLE 2. Factors Related to Noncompliance of Medication Regimen

Client Characteristic - Focused	Provider/Treatment - Focused	Environment/Situation - focused
Functional Impairments	Provider-Client Interaction	Access to Medication
* Decreased mobility	* Ineffective communication	* Lack of economic resources
Difficulty getting to pharmacy	* Lack of confidence in provider	* Containers that are difficult to open
Difficulty measuring liquid doses or breaking	* Lack of confidence in treatment	* Long distance to pharmacy
* Visual impairment	* Inadequate explanations of medication and medication regimens	* Labels that are difficult to read
Cannot read label		* Unclear directions
Cannot differentiate colors	* Absence of written material	
* Hearing impairment	* Infrequent monitoring and feedback	
Cannot hear instruction		
* Poor memory		
Cannot remember to take medications		

Client Characteristic – Focused	Provider/Treatment – Focused	Environment/Situation – focused
Perceptual Factors	Treatment Characteristics	Social Support
* Low perception of seriousness of condition	* Complexity of medications	* Living alone
* Low perception of susceptibility to condition	* Number of medications	* Nonsupportive attitdues of family members
* Low perception of efficacy of treatment	* Side effects of medications	
* Absence of symptoms	* Interactions between medications	
* Medication does not relieve symptoms	* Number of changes required in habits/lifestyle	
* High anxiety level	* Physician error (dose too high)	
* Fear of addiction to medications	* More than one provider	Treatment Setting
		* Many providers versus one provider
Educational Factors	* More than one pharmacy	* Home/community versus institutional
* Lacks understanding of medication regimen		
* Lacks knowledge about medications and regimen		

which providers can analyze the many possible variables that can interact and contribute to non-compliance.

Client-Focused Factors

Client characteristics focused factors are those which can be attributed to the patient, such as age, immobility, or lack of understanding regarding medication-taking. Demographic variables (i.e., age, sex, socio-economic status, education, religion, marital status, and race), when examined apart from other variables, have rarely been predictive of compliance with medical recommendations (Marston, 1970, p. 317). However, in a recent quality assurance project, LaLonde compared a group of men and a group of women (N = 121) randomly selected across five home care agencies in the state of Washington. Men took a higher percentage of their prescribed medication correctly in comparison to women (LaLonde, 1986). No data were available to provide an explanation of this finding.

Client characteristics that involve functional impairment have been documented as related to non-compliance. For example, mobility impairment from arthritis can create a barrier to being able to physically obtain or self-administer medications. Impairment in vision (e.g., label reading and color differentiation) is shown to be related to non-compliance. Similarly, deficits in hearing and short-term memory also interfere with taking the right drug at the right time in the right dose (Hurd & Butkovik, 1986; Lesage, Beck & Johnson, 1979; Tideiksaar, 1984).

Client characteristics that involve perceptions have been associated with non-compliance in many studies. Clients who perceive their diseases as being more serious were more likely to comply with medication regimens than were those who perceived their diseases to be less serious. In the same respect, clients who believed that their medical regimens would be effective were more likely to comply than were those who doubted the effectiveness. Another perception related to non-compliance was fear of addiction. Perceived absence of symptoms also contributed to non-compliance. High levels of anxiety and lack of understanding regarding medications/regimens related significantly to non-compliance (Christensen, 1978; Nelson, Stason, Neutra, Soloman, & McArdle, 1978; Tideiksaar, 1984; Marston, 1970; Haynes, Taylor, & Sackett, 1979; Cooper, Love, & Raffoul, 1982).

Provider/Treatment-Focused Factors

Provider/Treatment focused factors are those which involve either the interaction between provider and patient or characteristics of the treatment itself. Factors shown to be related to non-compliance in this category include: (a) ineffective communication reflected by client's level of understanding of medications and regimen, (b) client's lack of confidence in the provider, (c) lack of monitoring strategies and feedback, and (d) absence of written instructions (Lipton, 1982; Haynes, Taylor, & Sackett, 1979). In a study by Hulka, Cassell, Kupper, and Burdette, (1976), physician-patient pairs were examined to determine the extent to which non-compliance could be attributed to inadequate communications. When patients were given more and better information about their drugs, their compliance was significantly better. Evans and Spelman (1983) reported that compliance was improved by providing clients with more understandable information and by supplying written information, which resulted in increased knowledge of their regimen. They also found that the attitude of the doctor seemed to facilitate compliance. In another study reported by Christensen (1978), physicians were found to exhibit four compliance-gaining strategies: friendliness, medical authority, justification of medication use, and emphasis on the need to continue taking the medication. Extensive monitoring and follow-up activities also contributed to increasing compliance. Although the dynamics of the client-physician interaction requires more study, there is sufficient evidence to suggest that it is a key factor related to non-compliance.

Those factors related to non-compliance that involve characteristics of the treatment include: (a) manipulation of dosage, (b) complexity of treatment (i.e., multiple medications, varying dosages depending on the day, tapering dosages depending on the week), (c) number of side effects or perceived interactions, (d) amount of change required in lifestyle or habits, and (e) physician error (i.e., inaccurate prescription writing or inaccurate information giving)

(Lesage, Beck, & Johnson, 1979; Lipton, 1982; Evans & Spelman, 1983; Christensen, 1978; Nelson, Stason, Neutra, Soloman, & McArdle, 1978; Tideikassar, 1984; Marston, 1970; Haynes, Taylor, & Sackett, 1979).

Numerous studies have shown that complexity of the medication regimen has a negative impact on compliance. Christensen (1978) suggested that lack of compliance may be due to clients feeling confused and overwhelmed and that inconvenience resulted from the regimen inhibited compliance. LaLonde (1986), however, found no significant relationship between the frequency of doses or multiple medication regimens and taking medication as prescribed. Findings from this study were based on 121 patients served by five home care agencies in Washington state. The fact that these clients were being monitored by a home care agency, however, may have been a confounding variable.

Evans and Spelman (1983) reported that the high cost of medications could be a factor related to noncompliance. They suggest, however, that the literature reveals enough conflicting data to warrant more definitive research in this area. Marson (1970) reported that drugs with unpleasant side effects are likely to be omitted by clients. Cooper, et al. (1982) found that intentional non-compliance was more likely to occur in subjects who used two or more physicians and two or more pharmacies. Many treatment-related factors can contribute to non-compliance and, if detected, may be amenable to intervention in order to increase the probability of compliance.

Environmental/Situational-Focused Factors

Environmental/situational-focused factors contributing to noncompliance are quite specific. For example, childproof bottle caps have been associated with non-compliance because they are difficult for some people to open. Illegible labels have been indicated as contributing to non-compliance (Hurd & Butkovick, 1986; Lipton, 1982). Lack of family or social support seems to be related to noncompliance. Patients with family members who have nonsupportive attitudes were shown to be more non-compliant than those with supportive family members (Lipton, 1982; Evans & Spelman,

1983; Tideiksaar, 1984; Haynes, Taylor & Sackett, 1979). Treatment site has been shown to affect compliance. For example, patients treated in the hospital were shown to be more compliant than were those treated in a clinic or on an out-patient basis. Clients who use the services of more than one provider were less compliant than those who used one (Evans & Spelman, 1983; Cooper, Love, & Raffoul, 1982; Tideiksaar, 1984).

The socio-economic situation of clients may contribute to their ability to purchase medications, but research results seem to indicate that higher socio-economic status alone is not necessarily associated with higher rates of compliance (Marston, 1970).

A brief overview of three major groups of factors related to non-compliance is presented in Table 2. Although factors are listed separately, they frequently contribute in an interactive way to non-compliance and therefore must be considered in that respect. Therefore, it is essential to consider all factors in assessing medication compliance. Much remains unknown about why people do not take medications as prescribed. Furthermore, factors which have not been consistently related to non-compliance (i.e., income or educational level) may be important factors for individual clients. The following section comprises a review of recent research studies aimed at testing strategies to improve medication compliance in elderly people.

STRATEGIES FOR IMPROVING MEDICATION COMPLIANCE

The literature describing strategies for improving medication compliance was abundant, and included a variety of disciplines such as medicine and nursing, health services, health education, and other behavioral disciplines. The literature reviewed included research studies as well as review articles or general treatises on the subject. A summary of the major strategies is organized as follows: (a) strategies focused on the patient; (b) strategies focused on the provider, the patient/provider relationship, or the medication regimen; and (c) strategies focused on environmental factors. It must be recognized that there is considerable overlap between the categories and that the most effective overall strategy may include the best aspects of each.

Strategies Focused on the Client

The category of client focused strategies includes interventions aimed at changing behavior in the client. Educational approaches as well as counseling interventions were concerned. Strategies to assist clients to remember to take medications were also included in this category. Behavioral approaches were included in the patient/ provider relationship category because of their emphasis on interpersonal relationships.

Educational Strategies

The underlying assumption of studies focused on the transmission of information or instruction to the person who "needs to comply" with the medication regimen is that knowledge about disease or the specific medication regimen will lead to compliance with the prescribed medication regimen. The evidence is clear, however, that knowledge alone is not sufficient to ensure medication compliance (Haynes, Taylor, & Sackett, 1979; Richardson, 1986; Sands & Holman, 1985). In the elderly, possession of knowledge alone may be even less relevant in relation to medication compliance. Klein, German, McPhee, Smith, and Levine (1982) followed 545 patients discharged over a nine month period. Thirty-one percent were over the age of 65. Telephone interviews were conducted and questions were asked about knowledge of diagnosis and drug purpose, patterns of medication use, and other health behaviors. Results demonstrated that knowledge of disease process and medication purpose were significantly lower for elderly patients than for younger patients. However, compliance rates were similar for the two groups. There was no significant relationship between knowledge and medication compliance.

Recent studies of medication compliance in the elderly have incorporated written information or special counseling approaches into the educational intervention. Hammarlund, Ostrom, and Kethley (1985) surveyed elderly residents of a high-rise, low income housing unit regarding mediation behavior and provided on-the-spot teaching geared to identified problems. Residents also received written information about how to avoid medication problems and were offered formal classes as well as counseling about medication problems. Thirty nine residents with the greatest number of medication problems were reassessed after one year and found to have a 39 percent decrease in the number of medication behavior problems. There was no control group in this study. Norell (1979) randomized 82 glaucoma patients into a control group and an experimental group. The experimental group were shown a tape-slide show on the disease and its treatment and individuals received medication instruction tailored to individual life style and daily activities. The experimental group showed significantly higher levels of compliance as measured by the number of missed dosses of pilocarpine drops over a period of time. In another study, Garnett, Davis, McKenney, and Sterner (1981), assigned 82 patients taking a course of antibiotics to: (a) a control group, (b) a telephone call-back group, (c) a written and oral instruction group, and (d) a written and oral instruction plus call-back group. The three groups were significantly more compliant than the control group as determined by pill count. The follow-up telephone call group was equal to, but did not enhance written and oral consultation as a factor related to improvement in patient compliance.

Other studies have examined the impact of written information on medication compliance (Detullio, Eraker, Jepson, Becker, Fujimoto, Diaz, Loveland, & Stretcher, 1986; Lundin, Eros, Melloh, & Sands, 1980; Morris & Olins, 1984). The major conclusion from these studies was that written information is more effective if combined with individual verbal counseling about specific client medication problems. Morris and Halperin (1979) reviewed studies on written information and medication compliance prior to 1979. The major conclusion from this review also was that written information is best when accompanied by verbal consultation. The researchers cautioned, however, that most of the studies suffer from methodological problems and were not grounded in a theoretical framework.

Educational approaches that incorporated memory aids for patients having difficulty remembering to take medications were, in general, effective in improving medication compliance in the elderly. Wandless and Davie (1977) found that instruction plus a calendar reminder were more effective than instruction plus a medication card reminder. Ascione and Shimp (1984) also combined written and verbal information with memory aids into their educational interventions. They concluded that small amounts of specific information were more effective in teaching elderly patients and that forgetfulness to take medications was best improved by combining a reminder aid with verbal reinforcement. In this study, the medication reminder package was more effective than the calendar. Pavkov and Stephens (1981) also advocated the use of a memory reminder for nurses counseling clients about medication regimens.

Most of the educational programs reported in the literature were of short duration. Re-evaluation or reinforcement of behavior changes, therefore, was not generally incorporated as a component. However, in one study, Edwards and Pathy (1984) found that patients who were counseled about their medicines on the day of hospital discharge, and six days later by a health visitor showed significant improvement in compliance when compared to a group who did not receive the program. In addition, Harper (1984) recognized the importance of reinforcement of behavior change over time. She tested the effect of a medication self-care program for elderly hypertensive patients on knowledge of medicines, health locus of control, and self-care medication behaviors. The experimental program initially improved knowledge of medications, health locus of control and self-care behaviors. Follow-up over a six-month period, however, resulted in a diminutive effect on the variables.

The methods used in medication instruction for the elderly also had an impact on the success of the educational program. Kim and Gier (1981) compared slow-paced instruction (106 words per minute) to normal talking (159 words per minute). The slow-paced group had a greater gain from the pretest to the post-test and made significantly fewer errors to questions during the medication instruction than either the control or fast-paced group. Patients in both the control and the experimental group had difficulty recalling drug information 1.5 minutes after receiving it. Kim and Grier (1981) suggested the use of written information as well as verbal instruction to reinforce learning.

A popular misconception is that the elderly have more difficulty complying with medication regimens. Morisky, Levine, Green and

Smith (1982) tested the effects of a health education program on medication compliance related to hypertension control and compared a younger group with an elderly group of patients. The results of their study indicated that even though elderly patients have more chronic disease and received more complex therapies than younger patients, they demonstrated higher rates of medication compliance, appointment keeping and no difference in the proportion having their blood pressure under control at two year follow-up. They concluded that health education programs can be equally effective for an elderly population. Other studies support this conclusion (German, Klein, McPhee, & Smith, 1982; Skolnick & Eddy, 1984). In summary, there is strong support for the value of health education programs that employ a variety of methods to improve medication compliance in the elderly.

Psychological Strategies

Few studies specifically addressed the stress of living with long term chronic disease on patient medication compliance. Webb (1980) tested the effects of a vigorous, group patient education program versus a supportive, individualized psychosocial counseling approach in improving patient compliance. The psychosocial counseling focused on the concerns of the individual patient such as marital, family, employment, sexual and financial problems. One hundred twenty-three low income, rural, black hypertensive patients were assigned to the education group, the counseling group, or a control group. Neither additional patient education nor additional psychosocial counseling improved medication compliance significantly better than regular physician visits alone. The author speculated that because the counseling was focused on anxiety management related to individual life concerns, such counseling may be simply unrelated to health behaviors. It was suggested that persistent follow-up over time may be the key to improved compliance.

Strategies Focused on the Client/Provider Relationship or the Medication Regimen

The studies included in this section are of two major types. The first are those which focus on behavioral strategies or procedures that attempt to directly modify specific non-compliant behaviors.

Because behavioral strategies emphasize the importance of the client/provider relationship, they are appropriate for inclusion. The second group of studies are those related to modification of the medication regimen.

Basic to any behavioral strategy aimed at modifying specific noncompliant behaviors is a client/provider relationship in which there is mutuality of expectations; shared decision making; and mutual giving and receiving of feedback. Hilka, Cassell, Kupper, and Burdette (1976), in a study of factors associated with drug errors with a sample of 357 patients, found a significant relationship between good physician/patient communication and low level of all types of medication errors. When there was agreement between the physician and the patient about what the physician had told the patient about medications and the disease process, the rate of medication errors was low. Mutuality of expectations, therefore, is an important component of the relationship. Unmet expectations seem to lead to lowered compliance (Kasl, 1975).

The development of a mutual-participation relationship also contributes to successful behavioral strategies (Hanson, 1986). Brody (1980) suggested four steps for encouraging mutual-participation relationships: (a) establish active atmosphere by helping the patient feel valued and appreciated, (b) determine the patient's goals and expectation for treatment, (c) discuss the pros and cons of alternative evaluation and treatment approaches, and (d) elicit the patient's informed suggestions and preferences and negotiate any disagreements.

Assessing specific reasons for non-compliance were critical for planning behavioral intervention strategies. Important areas for assessment were beliefs about the treatment plan, extent to which the patient agrees with the plan and believes it can be carried out, and factors or barriers to carrying it out (Hanson, 1986). The importance of distinguishing between the intentionally and non-intentionally compliant patient was basic to determining the appropriate strategy.

Fedder (1982) emphasized the importance of an instrumental type of communication, defined as an explicit exchange in which the provider acts consistently and rationally. A specific interview guide has been successful in eliciting medication taking problems from the patients' perception (Atkinson, Gibson, & Andrews, 1978).

Contingency contracting has been cited as a promising intervention strategy for enlisting patient cooperation, particularly with regard to long-term treatment regimens. Janz, Becker, and Hartman (1984) defined contingency contracting as "specific negotiated agreement that provides for the delivery of positive consequences of reinforcers contingent on desirable behavior" (p. 165). The contracting process clearly outlines the responsibilities of both the client and the provider in relation to the goal that has been mutually defined. Thus, there was a transfer of power and accountability to the client. Successes attributed to this approach may be a function of the interpersonal process involved in the contracting process.

Janz, Becker, and Hartman (1984) reviewed 15 studies evaluating contingency contracting to increase compliance. Some of the behaviors targeted for change were smoking, weight change, renal disease regimen, and antihypertensive regimen. Conclusions from the review were: (a) contingency contracting produced short term positive effects; (b) contracts were easy to implement; (c) contracts were a useful addition to other strategies but may be best used in combination with other strategies; and (d) the "self-contract" was one the client managed entirely, with the health provider available for support and possible advice, and may be a better contract. Many of the 15 studies reviewed had conceptual and methodological difficulties, such as a lack of follow-up over time or absence of critical components of the contract design or process.

Self-monitoring was another strategy for assisting clients to focus on specific problematic behaviors. A self-monitoring program included observation, evaluation, and regulating of behavior (Young, 1986). For example, a patient may be given a calendar or card outlining when medications were to be taken. The patient then recorded each self administration on the calendar. The success of this approach depends, in large part, on effective communication patterns between the patient and provider (King & Peck, 1981; Haynes, Sackett, & Taylor, 1980). If the patient felt uncomfortable about discussing self-monitoring behavior, medication compliance may not be improved.

Tailoring was a strategy aimed at assisting the patient to integrate the taking of medications into activities of daily living. Tailoring required the provider to spend time with patients to identify events in their lives that occurred regularly and that could be used as cues for reminding patients to take medications. (King & Peck, 1981). Three types of cues have been identified by Schmidt (1979): (a) the direct cue — the patient left the medication bottle on the breakfast table and saw it when he or she ate breakfast; (b) the indirect cue — a novel cue or signal substituted for the medication (e.g., a note could be left on the refrigerator door); and (c) built in cue — self perpetuation such as putting the medication bottle in the shoe in the evening which will be a reminder to take it in the morning. The medication could be put on the pillow if it were to be taken in the evening, and then placed in the shoe.

Modification of the medication regimen by physicians is another strategy which may be helpful to increase medication compliance in the elderly. The results of some studies suggest that altering the number of doses of a medication to be taken during the day may contribute to improved compliance (Cohen, Gordon, Marlow, Belell, & Weathers, 1979; Norell, 1979, Norell, 1985). The notion of once-a-day dosing for medications has been strongly endorsed by the vice-president and general manager of G.D. Searle & Company (Bethune, 1985).

The number of medications taken and the complexity of the medication regimen have often been cited as factors related to medication non-compliance (Nelson, Stason, Neutra, Soloman, & McArdle, 1978; Lipton, 1982; Evans & Spelman, 1983; Tideiksaar, 1984; Marston, 1970; Haynes, Taylor, & Sackett, 1979). One approach to improving compliance, therefore, is simplifying the medication regimen by systematically reviewing the need for the medication and eliminating all those that are of questionable value (King & Peck, 1981; Haynes, Sackett, & Taylor, 1980).

Strategies Focused on the Environment

Strategies focused on the environment include those that changed or manipulated elements that were external to the patient. The strategies were of two major types. The first were studies that attempted to alter the medication bottle or the labeling of the bottle in order to facilitate ease in self-administration. The other major category was those interventions that focused on bolstering the social support system of the patient.

Bottle labeling of medications has been demonstrated to be important to patient understanding of proper administration. Elderly people may have additional problems with labels because of de creased visual acuity. A descriptive study of 60 elderly patients responsible for taking their own medications after discharge from the hospital revealed that 35 had problems reading their medication labels and did not have a clear understanding of the labeled directions (Zuccollo, G. & Liddell, H., 1985). Jumbo sized letters as well as choice and syntax of words used for directions need to be carefully selected.

Special packaging of medications, such as a unit dose with the date and time of day to be taken printed on the back, has been an effective and convenient method for the patient in carrying medications. However, special packaging has not always contributed to greater compliance. Becker, Glanz, Sobel, Mossey, Zinns, & Knott, (1986) tested the effects of special packaging (i.e., unit dose with the date and time of day to be taken) of antihypertensive medication on compliance and found no significant improvements in blood pressure control or compliance for patients receiving special medication.

It has been noted that elderly persons may have difficulty distinguishing between the green and blue tablets or between yellow and white tablets. The study suggests that health providers need to conduct a differentiation test using same-color and different-color pairs of the patient's medication. Assisting the patient to use other cues for differentiation, such as shape of bottle or shape of pill may be necessary.

Social Support Interventions

The evidence that a strong social support system is positively related to client compliance is well documented (Haynes, Taylor, & Sackett, 1979). Levy (1983) conducted a selective review and critique of studies that focused on manipulating the social support variable as the treatment program. Although the review did not focus specifically on medication compliance, the literature may suggest some helpful directions.

Four methods of bolstering social support were identified: (a) home visits, (b) significant other training, (c) structured reinforcement/contracting of significant others, and (d) support groups. In most of the studies reviewed, the concept of social support was poorly conceptualized. It was difficult, therefore, to draw clear conclusions on the specific effects of social support on medical regimen compliance. The studies reviewed, however, suggest that social support may be an important component in compliance and that further research efforts should be directed at operationalizing the concept of social support.

Gervasio (1986) reviewed selected literature indicating that family members may or may not be supportive, and may even constitute a barrier to compliance. Such factors as family members' sympathy and encouragement, their assumption of responsibility for the sick member's care, their willingness to make necessary changes in the environment, and the compatibility of unusual familial roles with the patient's new sick role, may contribute to the patient's level of compliance. Gervasio (1986) suggests that interventions to improve family support for patient compliance must include attempts to directly modify emotional, behavioral and cognitive aspects of the problems, rather than focusing on only one aspect. Research for comparing the relative efficacy of different familial interventions for fostering compliance does not exist at the present time.

DISCUSSION AND IMPLICATIONS
FOR INTERVENTIONS

Issues surrounding medication compliance in the elderly are complex and multifaceted. Problems associated with medication regimens include all the usual problems of compliance common to other age groups as well as the difficulties associated with age-related sensory, functional, and cognitive changes. For this reason, interventions focused on improving medication compliance need to consider a broad range of factors which may be contributing to medication problems.

It should also be mentioned that many problems related to medication regimens of elderly people may be due to inaccurate prescribing on the part of the physician. Many physicians are not aware of age-related changes that affect absorption and elimination of drugs. In addition, drug reactions and interactions can be compounded by the excessive use of alcohol and dietary practices.

The majority of the research studies testing an intervention program to improve medication compliance were fraught with conceptual and methodological problems. Perhaps one of the most serious problems related to the literature on medication compliance/non-compliance was the lack of conceptual clarity of what constitutes compliance or non-compliance. Many of the research studies were designed without differentiating between types of compliance problems. In addition, measures of compliance were not tested for reliability or validity. Many of the intervention strategies seemed to be planned without knowing the nature of the compliance problems of the subject group. This deficit was particularly true of the educational strategies. Few of the studies were grounded with a conceptual framework. Most of the studies were cross-sectional, one time designs. There were few longitudinal studies that measured the effects of the intervention over time.

In spite of conceptual and methodological problems, most of the research reported short-term improvements in compliance as a result of the intervention. Educational approaches were more effective if the educational program was geared to specific problems of the subjects and if more than one method of education was used (e.g., verbal plus written information). In addition, if the clients had memory problems or could not read labels or differentiate the color of the medicine, interventions focused on solving those specific problems tended to improve compliance. Gearing the pace of instruction to meet the need of elderly people also improved the educational program.

Strategies which specifically focused on assessing individual non-compliance problems and developing behavioral programs for effecting change also were reported as successful, at least for short periods of time. Behavioral strategies included a strong focus on developing mutual-participation relationships between the client and provider and a concerted effort to foster self-care practices of the client. Some of the behavioral studies indicated the importance of careful assessment to determine the nature of the non-compliance problem. Behavioral strategies could then be focused on individual problem behaviors. Those strategies which involved the client in goal setting, such as the contracting approach, or tailoring the program to specific client needs, demonstrated good results. Because the home care nurse interacts with clients on an individual basis and can involve the client in a mutual-participation relationship, the behavioral approaches may be helpful.

Finally, involving the client's family in supporting the maintenance of a medication regimen was reported as helpful for the overall success of a program. However, from the studies reviewed, the exact nature of the interventions used with the family members was unspecified. Because home care nurses interact with family members, the importance of including family members in the intervention program is worth considering.

The concept of compliance/non-compliance has been used in several studies and provides a framework for the development of assessment guides. For example, the importance of differentiating intentional from non-intentional non-compliance is critical in developing a change strategy. Non-intentional compliance problems may be resolved provided they can be detected through careful interviewing and planning of appropriate strategies focused on the specific reasons for the non-compliance. Intentional compliance problems, on the other hand, may be more difficult to change, particularly if the client's belief system is not compatible with the biomedical model.

Unfortunately, no interview guides were found in the literature for assessing intentional and non-intentional compliance. However, there were several other interview guides and medication history forms which may be developed into an assessment guide for differentiating the concept of intention versus non-intention. Once this determination is made, other interview guides can be developed to determine specific information about the particular medication compliance problems.

Before a determination can be made about individual client intentional or non-intentional non-compliance, it is necessary for the nurse to complete a comprehensive medication history or assessment. On the basis of these data, the nurse can determine factors related to individual client medication non-compliance behavior and can determine appropriate intervention strategies. For example, if the client has non-intentional, non-compliance problems such as lack of understanding of the medication regimen, the nurse can focus specifically an intervention program to assist the client in learning about the medication regimen. On the other hand, if the client is intentionally non-compliant, the intervention strategy will need to focus on obtaining additional data from the client regarding health beliefs about the disease process, efficacy of medication regimen, confidence in health providers, and adverse reactions.

The Comprehensive Medication Assessment Guide (see Attachment A) was developed to assess problems related to self-administration of medications that elderly home care clients may be experiencing. Factors derived from the literature related to medication non-compliance were used as a basis for developing the items in the medication guide (see Table 2).

DESCRIPTION OF THE COMPREHENSIVE MEDICATION ASSESSMENT INTERVIEW GUIDE

The purpose of the Comprehensive Medication Interview Guide is to assist health professionals in assessing underlying factors which may be contributing to unsafe/non-compliant practices related to medication self-administration by elderly clients. Although geared primarily for the home setting, the guide can also be used in other settings where the client is self-administering medications.

The Comprehensive Medication Assessment Interview Guide and the Individual Medication Assessment form (see Attachment A) were developed to be used together. The assessment form provides an opportunity for the nurse to record information based on the medication assessment.

The first five questions for the Interview Guide relate to checking the current medication bottles the client has in the home and comparing the labels with the physician orders on the agency chart. In addition, the nurse should note whether the medications are outdated, prescribed by more than one physician, or filled by multiple pharmacies. This is important information in determining discrepancies between what the client is taking and what the physician has ordered. The use of multiple physicians and pharmacies may contribute to multiple adversely interacting drugs being prescribed inadvertently.

Question 6 assess the client's knowledge about the purpose of the medication being taken. This is a safe place to start the assessment because clients generally like to talk about the medications they are taking. This assessment will provide the nurse with information about possible knowledge deficits that the client may have in relation to the purpose of particular drugs. However, before intervening with detailed information about the purpose of the medication, it is important to proceed to assess the beliefs, concerns, and problems related to their medication regimens.

Questions 7 and 8 focus on the client's perceptions and concerns about the medication regimen. Starting with these questions early in the interview encourages the client to share personal concerns and problems and will provide the interviewer with information useful in helping clients and families solve problems related to their medication regimens. It is obvious that if the client expresses concerns or fixed beliefs about medications, teaching about the purpose of the drug, the proper time, dose, frequency, special instructions may be premature. The concerns expressed by the client must first be resolved through mutual problem solving by the nurse, client, and family.

If the client does not express concerns about the medication regimen, then the nurse continues the medication assessment with questions 9 through 14. These questions assess the accuracy of the self-administration according to the prescriptive information: Is the client taking the medication according to the prescribed frequency, at the proper times, the correct amount and by the proper route? Does the client understand how and when to take PRN medications? Does the client understand the special instructions? Discrepancies can be noted and instructions clarified provided other concerns or problems are not contributing to the discrepancies. (For example, the client may not understand that the medication needs to be taken after eating food and simply explaining this fact may solve the problem. However, if the client is worried that the medication may cause an ulcer and does not want to take the medication at all, the strategy for problem solving may be quite different.)

Question 15 assesses other medications, drugs, and substances the client may be taking. In studying the teaching, coordination, and counseling activities of the 49 nurses who participated in testing the medication interview guide, 8 percent discussed over-the-counter drugs with their clients yet the importance of over-the-counter drugs and alcohol in contributing to drug interactions has been well documented in the literature.

Questions 16, 17, and 18 assess special physiological, psychosocial and environmental issues that may interfere with the elderly client's ability to manage the medication regimen. Possible functional and sensory deficits should be considered for all elderly clients as such deficits could interfere with medication self-administration. As indicated on the interview guide, having the client demonstrate the ability to open containers, read labels, or distinguish colors of drugs (particularly blue and green) may be appropriate with some clients.

In addition, if there is any indication that the client may be having problems remembering to take the medication (whether due to possible memory problems or depression) it is important to assess this area in depth. Questions 17 and 18 demonstrate questions which may elicit additional information about how the family and client are managing the medication regimen. In general, family members are intimately involved in either supporting and encouraging family members with their medication regimens or hindering or interfering with the medication regimen. The home care nurse must be able to assess family support and intervene when the family is not supportive or does not understand the goals for medication therapy.

Question 19 is a direct question aimed at assessing premature discontinuation of a medication. It is important to ask the client/or family because clients intentionally may decide to discontinue a medication if they have concerns about it or cannot afford the cost. This question is designed to elicit client concerns that have not been shared prior to this point in the interview.

Home storage of medications often presents problems for the client and family which may be related to lack of knowledge or inadequacy of facilities. It is important for the nurse to assess this area and differentiate any problems that may be evident.

Finally, questions 21 and 22 focus on obtaining information

about the quality of the client/provider relationships and whether or not the client feels comfortable in discussing concerns and beliefs about medications with other health providers. This places the nurse in a key position to facilitate communication with other providers.

Note that on Part III of the Individual Medication Assessment Form, there are four general diagnoses that summarize the client's medication-taking behavior. Based on the assessment data, the health professional decides in which general category the client fits. The first category is compliance with medication regimen. The client has no problems with the medication and is taking them according to prescription. The second category, non-compliance with medication regimen — unintentional, describes problems with medication which may be related to knowledge deficits, functional or sensory deficits, memory/cognitive, or psychosocial problems. A specific diagnosis can be made depending on the particular problem the client is experiencing. The third category, non-compliance with medication regimen — intentional, describes clients who make a deliberate decision to discontinue a medication due to health beliefs, side effects, or other concerns such as cost or fear of drug dependence. The fourth category is a combination of the previous three categories since some clients may be compliant with some of their medications but not with others.

FIELD TEST OF THE COMPREHENSIVE MEDICATION ASSESSMENT INTERVIEW GUIDE

The first objective of the field test of the comprehensive Medication Guide was to describe nursing activities of the total sample of 48 nurses related to medication assessment and intervention. The second objective was to test whether nurses who used the Comprehensive Medication Assessment Interview Guide performed significantly more nursing activities than nurses who used a standard assessment guide or no assessment guide. The final objective was to determine if significant differences occurred in categories of nursing activities reported by nurses who used the Comprehensive Medication Assessment Interview Guide as contrasted to nurses who used a standard assessment guide or no assessment guide. Specific categories of nursing activities included (1) communication/coordination with other providers, (2) counseling/discussion, (3) client/family teaching, and (4) direct nursing activities (see Table 3).

The design of the field study was a before-after treatment quasi-experimental design with two treatment groups and a control group. Each of the nurses in the treatment group used a medication assessment guide: (1) a standard assessment guide or (2) the Comprehensive Assessment Guide. The third group was a control group. This group did not use an assessment guide and staff members completed their medication assessment as usual. Data collection periods were one point in time.

Sample

Participants in the field test were 48 registered nurses drawn from six Medicare-certified home health care agencies in a Northwest metropolitan area. The 48 nurses were randomly assigned to the following groups: (1) Comprehensive Medication Interview Guide group, (2) standard medication assessment guide and (3) no assessment guide group. The groups therefore, were comprised of 16 nurses each.

Two-thirds (66.6 percent) of the sample were baccalaureate-prepared nurses with the remaining one-third equally divided between nurses who obtained their education in associate degree or diploma programs (16.7 percent) and nurses who received certificates or degrees beyond the baccalaureate level (16.7 percent). Forty-six percent of the sample had been in nursing practice for less than 10 years, whereas 54 percent had been in practice for 10 or more years. Fifty-four percent of the participants were full-time home health care nurses, whereas 46 percent practiced on a part-time basis. All study participants were volunteers from whom informed consent was obtained following both verbal and written explanation of the study. Human subjects approval for conducting the study was obtained through the University of Washington Human Subjects Committee.

TABLE 3. Specific Medication-Related Nursing Interventions

CATEGORY   PERCENT

COMMUNICATION/COORDINATION WITH OTHER PROVIDERS

Clarification/verification of medication orders................29
Exchange of information with M.D. or other provider...........29
Exchange of information with pharmacy, respiratory
  therapist, laboratory.......................................29
Contact to renew/update prescription or order/reorder medication....8
Contract with insurance companies, financial agencies..........0
Coordination/consolidation of multible pharmacies..............0

COUNSELING/DISCUSSION

Medication concerns or problems...............................31
Relative pros and cons of medication use, risk/benefit ratio....13
Client's beliefs regarding medication use.....................10
Negotiation of appropriate tailored administration 10
  regimen/routine
Discrepancies between prescription and practices...............8

CLIENT/FAMILY TEACHING

DIRECT NURSING ACTIVITIES

Procedure

Nurse participants were instructed to select one client from their current case load for whom they were planning to do an assessment of medication-taking behavior and who (a) was 65 years of age or over, and (b) had received at least one prior home visit. Group I nurses were instructed to use the Comprehensive Medication Assessment Guide in assessing medication-taking behavior of the client (see Attachment A). Group II nurses were instructed to use a standard form of medication assessment which included assessment of client medication-taking behavior in the following areas: (a) taking medications according to the prescribed frequency, (b) taking medications at the proper times, (c) taking the prescribed amount of the medication, (d) taking medication by the proper route, and (e) taking PRN medications for the proper reasons (see Attachment B). Group III nurses were instructed to complete a medication assessment with one of their clients without using a specific medication assessment form.

Within 48 hours after the visit to this client, nurse participants tape-recorded their responses to seven general questions regarding the nature of the medication-related assessments and interventions. Cassettes were then returned through the mail. Taped responses were coded into 35 specific categories by two investigators who listened to the cassettes together to maximize reliability of qualitative data through a process of consensual validation. The category and coding system (see Attachment C) was based on the Comprehensive Medication Assessment Guide.

Findings

Responses from the 48 nurses were combined for the initial analysis. The percentage of nurse participants who reported having performed each of the 35 specific medication-related assessments and interventions are presented in Table 3. None of the home health care nurse participants reported either (a) communication with insurance companies or financial agencies, or (b) coordination or consolidation of multiple pharmacies. Only 6 percent of the participants reported having created or assisted with sensory/functional aids for self-administration of medications by elderly clients, such as relabeling bottles with large print and prefilling pill containers or syringes. At the other extreme, 65 percent reported teaching clients or families about potential side effects, adverse reactions, and reportable signs and symptoms related to prescribed medications; 71 percent also reported teaching about the purpose of prescribed medications. Ninety-one percent of the participants reported specific medication-related plans for future nursing visits to the selected elderly home health care client.

Univariate statistical analyses by major categories (i.e., communication/coordination; counseling/discussion; client/family teaching; nursing activities) revealed no significant differences in reports of performance by the nurse demographic variables of educational preparation, number of years in nursing practice, employment status, or employment agency. However, multivariate analysis using a One-Sample Hotelling's T^2 with data from all 48 nurse participants combined, revealed significant mean differences among the first four categories, with counseling/discussion activities reported with the lowest mean frequency (X = .93, or less than one counseling/discussion activity per nurse for the selected visit) and client/family teaching reported with the highest mean frequency (X = 5.33, or over five teaching activities reported, on the average, by each nurse for the assessment visit) (see Table 4).

The data were examined further to determine if there were significant differences between the three groups (Group I, Comprehensive Medication Assessment; Group II, Standard Assessment; and Group III, no assessment) in the mean numbers of times nurses reported each of the 35 nursing activities. A Kruschal-Wallis ANOVA test was used for this analysis. The only significant difference for the 35 specific items was that Group III had significantly fewer reports of "teaching about special instructions" than Group I or Group II.

Data were also examined to determine if there were significant differences between the three groups in the mean number of times nurses reported items categorized in the four major categories: (a) communication/coordination, (b) counseling/ discussion, (c) teach-

TABLE 4. Mean Differences Among Major Categories of Medication-Related Nursing Interventions

Category Variable	Mean
Communication/Coordination	1.22
Counseling/Discussion	.93
Client/Family Teaching	5.33
Direct Nursing Activities	2.64

Hotelling's t Value	Approximate F	Hypothesized D.F.	Significance of F
7.789	85.689	4	0.00

ing, and (d) nursing activities. No significant differences were found among the three groups.

Discussion

When data were grouped and analyzed for all 48 nurses, findings of this study showed that home care nursing interventions were primarily concentrated within the realm of teaching. While information is certainly one important element in medication adherence, much of the teaching currently conducted by nurses is based on the questionable assumption that knowledge is directly translated into behavior. For example, studies have documented that teaching as a sole intervention strategy does not substantially increase medication adherence over time (Detullio, Eraker, Jepson, Becher, Fujimoto, Dias, Loveland, & Strecher, 1986; Sands, Holman, Skilnick, & Eddy, 1984). These studies suggest that other factors (e.g., attitudes, beliefs, financial concerns, physical limitations) are critical prerequisites to effective knowledge utilization, particularly with elderly clients.

Findings from the taped interviews of nurses in the present study indicated that nurses expressed frustration over the fact that clients were not following the nurses's instructions and teaching. However, the typical response to this frustration was *more* or repeated teaching rather than exploration and implementation of other intervention strategies (i.e., communication with other providers, counseling/discussion, monitoring and support activities).

More specifically, some of the *lowest* reported nursing interventions were (a) communication with insurance companies or financial agencies, (b) coordination or consolidation of multiple pharmacies, (c) discussion of discrepancies between prescriptions and practices, and (d) support activities related to sensory/functional deficits. These types of nursing interventions are based on assessing the specific individual needs and home situations and are fundamental in facilitating medication self-management by elderly clients. For example, teaching about medications purpose had little impact if a client cannot afford to purchase a prescription. Likewise, teaching about side effects or adverse reactions does not get to the root of the problem of a client purchasing prescriptions from multiple pharmacies. And teaching about a prn medication for pain may have little effect if the client does not believe that the medication will relieve the symptom. Finally, teaching about medication time, dose, route, etc., is fruitless if the client cannot even open the medication bottle. The findings suggest then, that home care nurses working with elderly clients do not always utilize the range of potential — and, in fact, indicated — nursing interventions for managing complex medication regimens. Communication with other providers, counseling/discussion, and direct nursing activities must supplement client/family teaching in fostering correct, self-administration of medications by elderly clients.

It was anticipated that nurses who used the Comprehensive Medication Assessment Guide would use a wider range of nursing activities in their interactions with clients. However, when data were analyzed by the treatment and control groups, only one significant difference was found among the groups in relation to the mean number reported for each of the 35 activities. Furthermore, no significant differences among the groups were found for the four major categories of nursing activities.

The lack of significant differences between the groups may be explained by the inability of nurses in Group I (Comprehensive Medication Assessment group) to grasp and use the assessment information suggested in the Comprehensive Medication Assessment Guide in the one home visit. Because the Guide is comprehensive, complex and detailed, perhaps nurses using the Guide would need to have studied the Guide carefully and have used it several times in order to focus on assessing areas of medication self-administration behavior not traditionally considered in medication assessment. Such areas as the client's concerns and problems related to medications, support and attitudes of family members in relation to the medication regimen, and functional and sensory deficits of the client which affect medication administration, require sophisticated interviewing skills. Group I nurses in this study had no inservice education in developing interview skills.

Should the study be repeated, it is suggested that nurses in Group I, the Comprehensive Medication Assessment group, receive a series of inservice education classes to become familiar with the Assessment Guide and to develop interviewing skills.

Agencies that use the Comprehensive Medication Assessment Guide may want to introduce the Guide to their staff by providing inservice education about the guide and suggested interviewing skills. A video-tape and training manual (Health Beliefs and Medications: Interviewing Techniques) are available through the Northwest Geriatric Education Center, Institute on Aging, JM-20, University of Washington, Seattle, WA 98195.

REFERENCES

Ascione, F. & Shimp, L. (1984). The effectiveness of four education strategies in the elderly. *Drug Intelligence and Clinical Pharmacy, 18*, 926-931.

Atkinson, L., Gibson, I., & Andrews, J. (1978). An investigation into the ability of elderly patients continuing to take prescription drugs after discharge from hospital and recommendation concerning improving the situation. *Gerontology, 24*(3), 225-234.

Becker, L., Glanz, K., Sobel, E., Mossey, J., Zinn, S., & Knott, K. (1986). A randomized trial of special packaging of antihypertensive medications. *The Journal of Family Practice, 22*(4), 357-361.

Bethune, D. (1985). View from the top. *American Druggist*, April, 30-35.

Blackwell, B. (1976). Treatment adherence. *British Journal of Psychiatry, 129*, 513.

Brody, D. (1980). The patient's role in clinical decision making. *Annals of Internal Medicine, 93*, 718-722.

Campbell, A., McCosh, L., & Reinken, J. (1983). Drugs taken by a population based sample of subjects 65 years and over in New Zealand. *New Zealand Medical Journal, 96*(732), 378-380.

Christensen, D. (1978). Review: Drug-taking compliance: A review and synthesis. *Health Services and Research*, Summer, 171-187.

Cohen, M., Gordon, R., Marlow, H., Bedell, J., & Weathers, L. (1979). A single-bedtime-dose self-medication system. *Hospital Community Psychiatry, 30*(1), 30-33.

Cooper, J., Love, D., & Raffoul, P. (1982). Intentional prescription nonadherence (non-compliance) by the elderly. *Journal of the American Geriatric Society, 30*(5), 329-333.

Department of Health and Social Security. (1978). *Health and Personal Social Services Statistics for England*. London: HMSO.

Department of Health and Social Security. (1982). *Health and Personal Social Services Statistics for England*. London: HMSO.

Detullio, P., Eraker, S., Jepson, C., Becker, M., Fujimoto, E., Diaz, C., Loveland, R., & Strecher, V. (1986). Patient medication instruction and provider interactions: Effects on knowledge and attitudes. *Health Education Quarterly, 13*(1), 51-60.

Ebert, N. (1980). The nursing process applied to the aged person receiving medication. In A. Yurick, S. Rob, B. Spier, & N. Ebert (Eds.). *The Aged Person and the Nursing Process* (pp. 483-484). New York: Appleton-Century-Crofts.

Edwards, M. & Pathy, M. (1984). Drug counseling in the elderly and predicting compliance. *The Practitioner, 228*, 291-300.

Evans, L. & Spelman, M. (1983). The problem of non-compliance with drug therapy. *Drugs, 25*, 63-76.

Fedder, D. (1982). Managing medication and compliance: Physician-pharmacist-patient interactions. *American Geriatrics Society, 30*(11) (Suppl.), 5113-5117.

Fletcher, S., Fletcher, R., Thomas, D., & Hamann, C. (1979). Patient's Understanding of prescribed drugs. *Journal of Community Health, 4*(3), 183-189.

Frisk, P., Cooper, J., & Campbell, N. (1977). Community-hospital pharmacist detection of drug-related problems upon patient admission to small hospital. *American Journal of Hospital Pharmacy, 34*(7), 738-742.

Garnett, W., Davis, L., McKenney, J., & Steiner, K. (1981). Effect of telephone follow-up on medication compliance. *American Journal of Hospital Pharmacy, 38*, 676-679.

Gerber, K. & Nehemkis, A. (Eds.). (1986). *Compliance: The Dilemma of the Chronically Ill*. New York: Spring Publishing.

German, P., Klein, L., McPhee, S., & Smith, C. (1982). Knowledge of and compliance with drug regimens in the elderly. *Journal American Geriatric Society, 30*, 568-571.

Gervasio, A. (1986). Family relationships and compliance. In K. Gerber & A. Nehemkis (Eds.). *Compliance: The Dilemma of the Chronically Ill*. (pp. 98-128). New York: Springer.

Hammarlund, E., Ostrom, J., & Kethley, A. (1985). The effects of drug counseling and other educational strategies on drug utilization of the elderly. *Medical Care, 23*(2), 165-170.

Hanson, R. (1986). Physician-patient communication and compliance. In K. Gerber & A. Nehemkis, (Eds.), *Compliance: The dilemma of the Chronically Ill* (pp 182-209). New York: Springer.

Harper, D. (1984). Medication for the elderly. *ANS, 6*(3), 29-46.

Haynes, R., Sackett, D., & Taylor, D. (1980). How to detect and manage low patient compliance in chronic illness. *Geriatrics*, 91-97.

Haynes, R., Taylor, D., & Sackett, D. (Eds.). (1979). *Compliance in Health Care*. Baltimore: The Johns Hopkins University Press.

Hulka, B., Cassell, J., Kupper, L., & Burdette, J. (1976). Communication and concordance between physicians and patients with prescribed medications. *American Journal of Public Health, 66*(9), 847-853.

Hurd, P. (1984). Aging and the color of pills. *New England Journal of Medicine*, January, 202.

Hurd, P., & Butkovick, S. (1986). Compliance problems and the older patient: Assessing functional limitations. *Drug Intelligence and Clinical Pharmacy, 20*(3), 228-230.

Janz, N., Becker, M., & Hartman, P. (1984). Contingency contracting to enhance patient compliance: A review. *Patient Education and Counseling,* 5(4), 165-178.

Kasl, T. (1975). Issues in patient adherence to health care regimens. *Journal of Human Stress,* September, 5-17, 48.

Kasper, J. (1982). *Prescribed Medications: Use, Expenditures and Source of Payment.* Data Preview 9, National Health Care Expenditure Study (DSHS Publication #PHS 82-3320). Washington, D.C.: U.S. Government Printing office.

Kendrick, R., & Bayne, J. (1982). Compliance with prescribed medication by elderly patients. *Canadian Medical Association Journal,* 127(10), 961-962.

Kim, K., & Grier, M. (1981). Pacing effects of medication instruction for the elderly. *Journal of Gerontological Nursing,* 7(8), 464-468.

King, N., & Peck, C. (1981). Enhancing patient compliance with medical regimens. *Australian Family Physician,* 10(12), 954-959.

Klein, L., German, P., Levine, D., Feroli, R., & Ardery, J. (1984). Medication problems among outpatients. A study with emphasis on the elderly. *Archives of Internal Medicine,* 144(6), 1185-1188.

Klein, L., German, P., McPhee, S., Smith, C., & Levine, D. (1982). Aging and its relationship to health knowledge and medication compliance. *The Gerontologist,* 22(4), 384-387.

Kofoed, L. (1985). Over the counter drug overuse in the elderly: What to watch for. *Geriatrics,* 40(10), 55-60.

Kovar, M. (1977). Health of the elderly and use of health services. *Public Health Report,* 92, 9-19.

Lalonde, B. (1986). *Quality Assurance Manual of the Home Care Association of Washington.* Seattle. Lalonde Research and Consultation. Mimeographed Report.

Lamy, P. (1982). Effects of diet and nutrition on drug therapy. *Journal of the American Geriatrics Society,* 30(11) (Suppl.), S99-S111.

Lamy, P. (1984). Hazards of drug use in the elderly. Common sense measures to reduce them. *Postgraduate Medicine,* 76(1), 50-53, 56-57, 60-61.

LeSage, J., Beck, C., & Johnson, M. (1979). Nursing diagnosis of drug incompatibility: A conceptual process. *Advances in Nursing Science,* 63-77.

Levy, R. (1983). Social support and compliance: A selective review and critique of treatment integrity and outcome measurement. *Social Science and Medicine,* 17(18), 1329-1338.

Lipton, H. (1982). Commentary: the graying of America: Implications for the pharmacist. *American Journal of Hospital Pharmacy,* 39(1), 131-135.

Lundin, D. (1978). Medication taking behavior of the elderly: A pilot study. *Drug Intelligence Clinical Pharmacy,* 12(9), 518-522.

Lundin, D., Eros, P., Melloh, J., & Sands, J. (1980). Education of independent elderly in the responsible use of prescription medications. *Drug Intelligence Clinical Pharmacy,* 14(5), 335-342.

Marston, M. (1970). Compliance with medical regimens: A review of the literature. *Nursing Research,* 19(4), 312-323.

Mathews, P., & Hingson, R. (1977). Improving patient compliance. *Medical Clinics of North America*, *61*, 879-889.

McKenney, J., & Harrison, W. (1976). Drug related hospital admissions. *American Journal Hospital Pharmacy*, *33*(8), 792-795.

Morisky, D., Green, L., & Levine, D. (1986). Concurrent and predictive validity of a self-reported measure of medication adherence. *Medical Care*, *24*(1), 67-74.

Morisky, D., Levine, D., Green, L., & Smith, D. (1982). Health education program effects on the management of hypertension in the elderly. *Archives of Internal Medicine*, *142*(1), 1835-1838.

Morris, L. & Halperin, H. (1979). Effects of written drug information on patient knowledge and compliance: A literature review. *American Journal of Public Health*, *69*(1), 47-52.

Morris, L. & Olins, A. (1984). Utility of drug leaflets for elderly consumers. *American Journal of Public Health*, *74*(2), 157-158.

Nelson, C., Stason, W., Neutra, R., Soloman, H., & McArdle, P. (1978). Impact of patient perceptions on compliance with treatment for hypertension. *Medical Care*, *16*(2), 893-906.

Norell, S. (1979). Improving medication compliance: A randomised clinical trial. *British Medical Journal*, *1*(6057), 359-361.

Norell, S. (1981). Monitoring compliance with pilocarpine therapy. *American Journal of Ophthamology*, *92*(5), 727-731.

Ostrom, J., Hammarlund, E., Christensen, D., Plein, J., & Kethley, A. (1985). Medication usage in the elderly population. *Medical Care*, *23*(2), 157-164.

Ouslander, J. (1981). Drug therapy in the elderly. *Annals of Internal Medicine*, *95*, 711-722.

Parkin, D., Henney, C., Quirk, J., & Crooks, J. (1976). Deviation from prescribed drug treatment after discharges from hospital. *British Medical Journal*, *2*(6037), 686-688.

Pavkov, J. & Stephens, B. (1981). Special considerations for the community-based elderly. *Geriatric Nursing*, *2*(6), 422-428.

Quality Assurance Manual of the Home Care Association of Washington (1986). Lalonde Research and Consultation. Seattle, WA: Lalonde, B.

Richardson, J. (1986). Perspectives on compliance with drug regimens among the elderly. *The Journal of Compliance in Health Care*, *1*(1), 33-45.

Roe, D. (1986). Drug-nutrient interactions in the elderly. *Geriatrics*, *41*(3), 57-74.

Sands, D. & Holman, E. (1985). Does knowledge enhance compliance? *Journal of Gerontological Nursing*, *11*(4), 464-468.

Schmidt, J. (1979). A behavioral approach to patient compliance. *Postgraduate Medicine*, *65*(5), 219-224.

Sklonick, B. & Eddy, J. (1984). Medication compliance and the aged: An educational challenge. *Educational Gerontology*, *10*, 307-315.

Simonson, W. (1984). *Medications and the Elderly: A Guide for Promoting Proper Use*, Aspen Systems Corporation, Rockville, Md.

Smith, M. & Sharpe, T. (1984). A study of pharmacists' involvement in drug use by the elderly. *Drug Intelligence Clinical Pharmacy, 18*(6), 525-529.

Squire, A., Goldman, M., Kupersmith, J., Stern, E., Fuster, V., & Schweitzer, P. (1984). Long term anti-arrhythmic therapy. Problem of low drug levels and patient noncompliance. *American Journal of Medicine, 77*(6), 1035-1038.

Tideiksaar, R. (1984). Drug noncompliance in the elderly. *Hospital Physician, 3*, 92-101.

Vestal, R. (1982). Pharmacology and aging. *Journal of the American Geriatric Society, 30*(3), 191-198.

Vestal, R. (1984). *Drug Treatment in the Elderly.* Boston: ADIS Health Science Press.

Wade, B. & Bowling, H. (1986). Appropriate use of drugs by elderly people. *Journal of Advanced Nursing, 11*(1), 47-55.

Wade, B. & Finlayson, J. (1983). Drugs and the elderly. *Nursing Mirror, 156*(18), 17-21.

Wandless, I. & Davie, J. Can drug compliance in the elderly be improved? *British Medical Journal, 1*(6057), 359-361.

Webb, P. (1980). Effectiveness of patient education and psychosocial counseling in promoting compliance and control among hypertensive patients. *Journal of Family Practice, 10*(6), 1047-1055.

Young, M. (1986). Strategies for improving compliance. *Topics in Clinical Nursing*, January, 30-38.

Zuccollo, G. & Liddell, H. (1985). The elderly and the medication label: Doing it better. *Age and Aging, 14*(6), 71-376.

ATTACHMENT A. Interview Guide for Comprehensive Medication Assessment of Elderly Clients

Interview Question	Guides and Rationale
PART I	
1-5 What medications are you taking now?	1-5 A. Have client or family member collect together all medications and bring to you.
	B. Check instructions on label with orders on chart. Check date obtained and expiration dates. Check for multiple prescribing physicians and multiple pharmacies. For any discrepancies or problems noted, probe further for possible reasons.
6. Can you tell me what this medication is supposed to do for your condition?	6. To assess client's knowledge and understanding about the purpose of the prescribed medication and client's need for information.
7. Do you think this medication is working for you?	7. To assess client's beliefs about the efficacy of the prescribed medication.
8. Do you have any concerns about taking this medication?	8. To assess client's concerns about the costs/risks related to the prescribed medications.
	A. High cost of medications
	B. Fear of drug dependence
	C. Adverse or side effects/drug interactions
	D. Ability to obtain (e.g., difficulty getting to pharmacy, lack of transportation)
	E. Interference with lifestyle (e.g., eating habits, religious beliefs, sleep patterns)
	F. Other (specify)

For Questions 9-13, probe for specified reasons if discrepancies are noted between prescribed instructions and client's practices.

9. How many times during the day do you take this medication?

To assess if the client is taking the medication according to the prescribed frequency.

10. When do you take this medication? At what hours or times of the day?

To assess if the client is taking the medication at the proper times.

11. How much of the medication do you take?

To assess if the client is taking the prescribed amount (dose) of the medication.

12. How are you taking this medication?

To assess if the client is taking the medication by the proper route, especially for creams, liquids, and topicals.

13. Are there any medications that you take only as necessary or periodically?

To assess if the client is taking PRN medications appropriately and for the proper reasons.

14. Are there any special instructions or precautions you follow in taking this medication?

To assess client's comprehension of and adherence to special instructions for self-administration of medications (e.g., don't drive, take only with food).

59

Interview Question	Guides and Rationale
PART II	
15. What other medications/ drugs/substances are you taking other than the prescription medications we've been discussing?	15. To assess client use of: A. Over-the counter drugs B. Alcohol C. Vitamins/Nutritional Supplements D. Other
16. Do you have any of the following difficulty that interfere with you taking your medications: Opening containers? Breaking tablets? Giving eye drops? Handling syringes? Reading labels? Distinguishing color of pills?	16. To assess for functional and sensory impairments that may cause barriers to self-administration of medications. For suspected deficits, ask client to: Open container Read label to you
17. Many people have some difficulty in remembering to take their medications. Are there times when you have difficulty remembering to take your medications? Or are there times when you just don't want to remember to take your medications?	17. To assess for cognitive/memory or psychological problems (e.g., depression) which may interfere with remembering to take their medications.

60

18.	Do you have some methods (tricks) you use to help you plan or remember to take your medications? Describe what happened the last time you forgot to take your medication. What do you do when you forgot to take a dose? Is there anyone here in your home (e.g., spouse) or someone close by who can encourage you or help you to remember to take your medication?	To assess for family/lifestyle or social problems which may interfere with self-administration of medications.
19.	Are there any medications that you have stopped taking altogether?	To assess for premature medication discontinuation by the client. Possible reasons: A. Absence of symptom or symptom improvement B. Medication fails to improve or relieve symptom C. High cost of medication (expense) D. Fear of drug dependence E. Adverse or side effects F. Difficulty in obtaining medications G. Interference with lifestyle H. Lack of confidence in physician I. Lack of proper instruction about medication regimen J. Other (specify):

Interview Question		Guides and Rationale	
20.	Where do you store (or keep) your medications?	20.	To assess proper storage of medications (e.g., determine if medications requiring refrigeration are stored in refrigerator).
21.	When you have problems with or concerns about your medications, do you feel free (comfortable) in calling or talking to your physician?	21.	To assess quality of the client/provider relationship. If client does not feel comfortable, additional description of the client/physician relationship should be requested.
22.	Is there anyone else you can talk to about your medication concerns or problems? Family, friends, pharmacist?	22.	To assess client's choice of support persons regarding medication problems. Are they appropriate (e.g., knowledgeable, reliable) for addressing concerns, giving sound advice?

ATTACHMENT B. Individual Medication Assessment Form

PART I

Fill out the Individual Medication Assessment Form for each medication the client is taking.

1. Name of medication(s)
    1 _____   2 _____   3 _____

    4 _____   5 _____   6 _____

    7 _____   8 _____   9 _____

    10_____   11 _____   12 _____

2. Are medication instructions the same on the bottle and chart?   Yes   No

3. Are medications old or outdated?   Yes   No

4. Are medications prescribed by more than one physician?   Yes   No

5. Are medications obtained from more than one pharmacy?   Yes   No

For the items below, circle either "Yes" or "No" for each medication the client is taking. Include comments as indicated.

		YES					NO		
		med	med	med	med		med	med	med	med
6.	Does the client have a correct understanding	1	2	3	4		1	2	3	4
	about the purpose of the medication?	5	6	7	8		5	6	7	8
	Comments if "No":	9	10	11	12		9	10	11	12
7.	Does the client believe that the medication is	1	2	3	4		1	2	3	4
	helping his/her condition?	5	6	7	8		5	6	7	8
	Comments if "No":	9	10	11	12		9	10	11	12
8.	Does the client have any concerns about or problems	1	2	3	4		1	2	3	4
	regarding taking the medication?	5	6	7	8		5	6	7	8
		9	10	11	12		9	10	11	12

If "YES" check which of the following apply: YES   NO

A.   High cost of medications   _____   _____
B.   Fear of drug dependence   _____   _____
C.   Adverse or side effects/reactions   _____   _____
D.   Ability to obtain medications   _____   _____
E.   Interference with lifestyle   _____   _____
F.   Other (specify):

9.	Is the client taking the medication according to	1	2	3	4		1	2	3	4
	the prescribed frequency?	5	6	7	8		5	6	7	8
	Comments if "No":	9	10	11	12		9	10	11	12

		YES				NO			
		med	mod	med	med	med	med	med	med
10.	Is the client taking the medication at the proper times?	1	2	3	4	1	2	3	4
		5	6	7	8	5	6	7	8
	Comments If "No":	9	10	11	12	9	10	11	12
11.	Is the client taking the prescribed amount (dose) of the medication?	1	2	3	4	1	2	3	4
		5	6	7	8	5	6	7	8
	Comments If "No":	9	10	11	12	9	10	11	12
12.	Is the client taking the medication by the proper route?	1	2	3	4	1	2	3	4
		5	6	7	8	5	6	7	8
	Comments If "No":	9	10	11	12	9	10	11	12
13.	Is the client taking PRN medications appropriately and for the proper reasons?	1	2	3	4	1	2	3	4
		5	6	7	8	5	6	7	8
	Comments If "No":	9	10	11	12	9	10	11	12
14.	Is the client following special Instructions for taking medications?	1	2	3	4	1	2	3	4
		5	6	7	8	5	6	7	8
	Comments If "No":	9	10	11	12	9	10	11	12

PART II

		YES	NO
15.	Is the client taking other medications or substances which may interact with prescribed medications?	_____	_____

If "YES" check which of the following apply:

A.	Over-the-counter drugs	_____
B.	Alcohol	_____
C.	Vitamins	_____
D.	Other (specify)	

		YES	NO
16.	Does this client have functional or sensory impairments which may interfere with self-administration of medications?	_____	_____

YES   NO

If "YES" check any which apply:

A. Manual dexterity problems (e.g., cannot open containers or break tablets, cannot administer eye drops, cannot handle syringe).

B. Visual problems (e.g., cannot read label, distinguish color of pills) _____

C. Other (specify):

17. Does this client have cognitive/memory or psychological problems which may interfere with self-administration of medications? _____ _____

If "YES" check any which apply:

A. Cognitive/memory impairment _____
B. Depression _____
C. Other (specify):

18. Does this client have lifestyle or social problems which may interfere with self-administration of medications? _____ _____

If "YES" check any which apply:

A. Lack of assistance or support from family and/or friends _____
B. Lack of routine for medication regimen and/or other schedule conflicts _____
C. Other (specify):

19. Has this client stopped taking prescribed medication(s) without instructions or orders to discontinue? _____ _____

If "YES" check any reasons which apply:

A. Absence of symptom or symptom improvement _____
B. Medication fails to improve or relieve symptom _____
C. High cost of medication (expense) _____
D. Fear of drug dependence _____
E. Adverse or side effects _____
F. Difficulty in obtaining medication(s) _____
G. Interference with lifestyle _____
H. Lack of confidence in physician _____
I. Lack of proper instruction about medication regimen _____
J. Other (specify):

	YES	NO
20. Does the client store medication properly?	-----	-----
Comments If "YES":		

21. Does the client have difficulty in discussing problems related to medications with his/her physician or primary provider?   -----   -----

Comments If "YES":

22. Does the client discuss problems related to medications with anyone else (e.g., family, friends, pharmacist)?   -----   -----

Comments If "YES":

PART III

Based on your assessment of this client, check the nursing diagnosis which best summarizes this client's medication-taking practices:

-----   Compliance with medication regimen
(Client has accurate knowledge and understanding of medication regimen, concurs with medication regimen, and generally takes medications as prescribed).

-----   Noncompliance with medication regimen, Unintentional.
(Client has inaccurate/inadequate knowledge and understanding of medication regimen or is not adhering to medication regimen due to physical, psychological, or social barriers).

-----   Noncompliance with medication regimen, Intentional
(Client has accurate knowledge and understanding of medication regimen and no physical, psychological, or social barriers to medication self-administration but has made a deliberate decision not to take medications as prescribed).

-----   Combination of compliance, unintentional noncompliance, and/or intentional noncompliance, depending on the specific drug. Specify:

ATTACHMENT C. Nurse Tape Interview Coding Form

COMMUNICATION/COORDINATION WITH OTHER PROVIDERS/SYSTEMS	
Clarification or verification of medication orders with M.D., pharmacist, hospital	
Telephone call to M.D. to renew/update prescription or call to pharmacist to order/reorder medication	
Exchange of information about client's attitudes, beliefs, med-taking practices, or condition (e.g., adverse reactions, side effects) with M.D. or primary provider	
Exchange of information with other sources (i.e., pharmacy, respiratory therapist, lab.	
Communication with insurance companies, financial agencies	
Coordination/consolidation of multiple pharmacies	

TEACHING	
Teaching about purpose of prescribed meds	
Teaching about prescribed frequency of meds	
Teaching about prescribed medication time	
Teaching about prescribed medication dose	
Teaching about prescribed medication route	
Teaching about PRN medication use	
Teaching about special instructions for self-administration of meds (e.g., take with food, avoid driving)	

NURSING ACTVITIES	
Physical/physiological monitoring for specific medication effects (e.g., takes pulse, B.P., resp; ogtains urine or blood tests)	
In-depth or formal psychosocial monitoring (e.g., cognitive/memory testing, family evaluation social network analysis)	
Obtains or delivers meds	
Administers or prepares meds (e.g., includes drawing up injections, breaking pills)	
Creates or assists with medication reminders (e.g., writes out time schedule/calendar, fills weekly pill container	

COUNSELING/DISCUSSION	
Counseling/discussion about client's beliefs regarding medication use	
Counseling/discussion about medication concerns/problems	
Counseling/discussion about relative "pros and cons" of medication use; relative risk/benefit ratio	
Discussion/exploration of discrepancies between prescription and practices	
Counseling/discussion negotiation of appropriate tailored administration regime or routine with client and/or family	
counseling/discussion, general -- nonspecific	

TEACHING	
Teaching about potential side effects, adverse reactions, self-monitoring, reportable signs and symptoms	
Teaching about med storage	
Teaching, general - nonspecific	

NURSING ACTIVITIES	
Mobilizes social resources (e.g., reminders/assistance/ periodic check-ups by family member, neighbor	
NURSING DIAGNOSIS, general (nonspecific)	
NURSING DIAGNOSIS, specific compliance v. noncompliance; intentionality v. nonintentionality	
NURSING PLANS, general (nonspecific)	
NURSING PLANS, specific (plans for follow-up assessment, further monitoring, future interventions	

Chapter III

Tailoring Teaching to the Elderly in Home Care

Martha Iles Worcester, PhC
Principal Author

Ann Loustau
Consultant

Kathleen O'Connor, MA
Editing

SUMMARY. This paper provides a brief overview of teaching and learning principles common to all adult learners and then discusses the latest research findings and their implications for adapting teaching materials and methods for the elderly. Sensory abilities, cognitive abilities, motor dexterity, developmental tasks, cohort influences, and the current situation in which the older person exists are included. Summary tables of key information are provided throughout the text for easy reference. Guides for assessment of the older adult, aids for evaluating educational materials, and a list of resources for teaching the older adult are provided in the appendix.

This paper is a portion of the material developed by the project staff of the Elderly Home Care Project, Principal Investigator, Barbara J. Horn. Funded by Fred Meyer Charitable Trust. Sponsoring agency: University of Washington, Department of Community Health Care Systems, Seattle, WA 98195.

INTRODUCTION

Background and Purpose

This paper was written in response to a need identified by the staff of home care agencies that participated in the Elderly Homecare Project (Horn, 1986). The project's purpose was to promote independence in the elderly by providing information and developing assessment and teaching materials that could be used by staff in home care agencies to support the elderly living at home. As part of that project a survey was conducted among 178 medicare certified agencies in the Northwest region of the United States to identify problems occurring as a result of earlier hospital discharge of the elderly. Of the top nine problems identified by the 118 agencies who responded, four problems included a teaching component. The problems with teaching components and the percentage of agencies who reported them were:

Teaching patients and their families

1. management of medication regimens...............90.9%
2. management of diabetes 88.6%
3. care of surgical wounds 83.0%
4. the care and administration of IV therapies..........81.8%

Because teaching the elderly has some aspects that are unique, it was decided to develop a separate state-of-the-art paper dealing with those unique aspects. Subsequent papers on the specific problems cited above were developed later to adapt teaching approaches for the elderly by applying the strategies developed in this paper.

Overview of Content

This paper is organized into three parts. The introduction includes the purpose of the paper and a brief review of the teaching and learning process common to all adult learners. The second part summarizes research on changes due to aging that most affect learning and analyzes implications of the changes for teaching elders. The third and final section summarizes basic principles to guide teaching and learning of the elderly in the home care setting. An appendix provides recommendations for teaching, learning and resources for home care agencies.

Importance of Teaching Older Adults

Given the current changing health care system, teaching self-care techniques is imperative. Shorter hospital stays shift more responsibility for client care to a home care setting. Teaching is difficult since it occurs at a time when the elderly client is recovering from an acute illness and beginning to manage on-going chronic illnesses. Accompanying this adjustment is the very limited number of reimburseable home visits. Visits for educational purposes have rigid reimbursement criteria and require documentation (Pesznecker, Horn, Werner, & Kenyon, 1987). Despite the increasing numbers of the elderly in our society and shorter lengths of hospital stay, funding for home care has not increased. Thus, teaching the elderly, as well as the family and friends who support them in the community, is critical to maintaining the health and well-being of our aging society.

Teaching, Learning, and Evaluation

Teaching

Teaching is a process of assisting persons to learn information and incorporate new knowledge and behavior into everyday life. It involves *assessing* the learner's abilities; *planning* and deciding with the learner what needs to be taught; *implementing* methods and resources that will maximize learning; and *evaluating* with the learner if goals have been reached (Smith, 1987a & c). Teaching is not simply relaying information. It includes the four steps of assessing, planning, implementing, and evaluating all of which are familiar processes to home care personnel who use the same four steps when developing client care plans.

Learning

Learning, on the other hand, is done by the person being taught. It entails the acquisition of new knowledge, behaviors, and beliefs. The three types of learning that occur are: (a) cognitive – acquisition of knowledge; (b) psychomotor—acquisition of new skills or behaviors; and (c) affective—acquisition of new beliefs or values (Bloom et al., 1956; Krathwohl, Bloom & Masia, 1964; Reilly, 1980; & Simpson, 1972).

Evaluation

Evaluation is the process that determines learning has occurred. It parallels the three types of learning discussed above and is reflected in: (a) ability to recall and explain the information taught; (b) correct performance of necessary actions for health and illness care and change in health status; and (c) changes in the learner's attitudes and beliefs that reflect valuing of the information or behavior respectively (Redman, 1984). Evaluation is based on accomplishing goals that are set with the learner.

Clinicians are familiar with determining a care plan with clients. Use of terms that are helpful in writing goals or objectives in each of the three areas of learning are provided along with sample care plan (see Appendix A).

Important Considerations for Learning

Learning is influenced by many factors. A review of those factors is presented in Table 1. The factors include: (a) teacher considerations; (b) learner considerations; (c) interactions between teacher and learner; and (d) situational influences.

Teacher considerations are those over which the teacher has the most control. Learner considerations are those that are part of the learner's life and experience. Interactions between the teacher and learner are factors that enhance mutual agreement on learning needs and desired outcomes. Situational influences are those factors external to the teacher or learner that are likely to impede or enhance learning. The list presented in Table 1 is compiled from a wide variety of sources including Botwinick (1984), Redman (1984), Reilly (1980), and Smith (1987b).

Although the considerations presented are applicable for all adult learners, how they are implemented will vary based on the type of setting, the number of people being taught and on the age and health of the learner. In order to determine what considerations are most

TABLE 1. Important Conditions for Learning

A. Teacher considerations:

  1. The learner's current knowledge, experience, and readiness for learning are assessed .
  2. An environment for learning is created that is free of distractions.
  3. Illustrations drawn from the life or knowledge of the learner are used.
  4. Teaching is timed close to when it will be applied.
  5. Several modalities are used: verbal, visual, and practice of using the knowledge.
  6. Review of material and feedback is provided.
  7. Goals and objectives of learning take into account the learner's wishes and needs.

B. Learner considerations:

  1. There is attention given to the material to be learned.
  2. There is motivation to learn.
  3. There is adequate physical and mental ability to learn.
  4. New learning or behavior can be incorporated into already established life patterns.
  5. There is a positive attitude toward learning.
  6. There is enough freedom from internal stresses that might inhibit learning.
  7. There is openness to alternatives and to new ideas.

C. Interactions between the learner and teacher:

  1. There is credibility of the teacher to the learner.
  2. There is rapport between teacher and learner.
  3. The teacher is sensitive to the learner's needs.
  4. There is agreement between the teacher and learner on what is important to learn and in what sequence.
  5. There is respect shown for what the learner already knows and for the learner's life style.

D. Situational considerations

  1. The setting is conducive to learning (absent of competing stimuli for attention).
  2. There are not other things going on in the learner's life that take priority over learning the information presented.
  3. The teaching method and content have been adapted to the setting.
  4. Persons important to the learner encourage and support the new knowledge, behaviors, and beliefs or values.

important for the older adult learner in the home setting, the clinician or teacher must first become aware of the characteristics and life situations of the elderly that most affect learning.

RESEARCH FINDINGS AND IMPLICATIONS FOR TEACHING OLDER ADULTS

Characteristics of Research Populations

In order to interpret correctly the results of research studies that follow, three characteristics of the samples in research populations should be kept in mind. First, studies that are done to compare the elderly with younger populations most commonly use a sample of people who are healthy (Hoyer & Plude, 1980), so that "age" differences can be determined rather than differences due to illness.

Second, the variability found within older populations participating in research studies is greater than the variability found in younger age groups. The variability is both within the individual and between individuals. "Within" means that an older person has greater differences from one testing period to the next. "Between" refers to the range of differences between one person and other persons in the older population. The range of difference "between" is greater among the elderly than it is for younger populations (Willis and Baltes, 1980). Home care staff should note these differences because it means that individual assessment for teaching adaptations is even more important for older clients.

The third characteristic of older research populations is that most studies categorize the elderly over 65 into one age group. However, persons at ages 65-74, 75-84, and 85 and over are quite different. Table 2 illustrates the extent of the variability among these age groups.

The research applicable to the older adult's ability to learn will address differences between the younger and older populations in the following areas: (a) sensory changes in vision and hearing; (b) cognitive differences related to intelligence tests, perception, processing, and response time; (c) motor dexterity differences; (d) developmental differences; (e) historical and cohort differences; and (f) situational differences.

TABLE 2. Variability of the Aged in Three Age Groupings

ITEM	Source	PERCENTAGE OCCURRENCE WITH AGE		
		65 to 74	75 to 84	85+
Cannot read with glasses	(1)	10%	14%	46%
Cannot hear normal voice	(1)	12%	15%	25%
Cognitive impairment	(2)	4%		25%
Needs assistance with walking	(3)	4%	8%	26%
Needs assistance with instrumental activities of daily living*	(3)	6%	14%	40%
Needs assistance with basic activities of daily living*	(3)	5%	11%	35%
Educational levels	(1)			
0 to 8		30%	41%	48%
high school		32%	23%	20%
13 +		20%	18%	13%
Income below poverty (1985)	(4)	12%	23%	31%
Living situations	(1)			
live alone		24%	38%	45%
with spouse		58%	48%	32%
3 or more in house		15%	12%	19%

* Instrumental Activities include items such as shopping, transportation, handling finances. Basic Activities include walking, bathing, dressing, eating, toileting, and getting out of a chair or bed. Reference sources are (1) Huntley, Brock, Ostfeld, Taylor, & Wallace, 1984: (2) Spar, 1982: (3) Feller, 1983: (4) US Department of Commerce ,1985, p. 97.

Sensory Changes

Vision

Research Findings. Vision difficulties increase with age. Persons who cannot read newsprint even with glasses comprise ten percent of the population at ages 65-74, fourteen percent at 75-84, and forty-six percent at 85 and over (Huntley, Brock, Ostfeld, Taylor & Wallace, 1984). With aging, the crystalline lens becomes less transparent, increases in thickness, and is less able to transmit and refract light. Yellowing of the lens decreases the quality of light perception. Sensitivity to colors at the upper end of the visual spectrum (yellow, orange and red) can be distinguished more easily than colors at the lower end of the visual spectrum (blue, green and violet). The pupil area becomes smaller and reduces the quality of light reaching the retina resulting in reduced visual acuity and reduced accommodation to distance and darkness (Hallburg, 1976; Botwinick, 1984). In addition, there are changes in the visual field. Sensitivity to light changes with decreases in the upper half of the visual field more than in the lower half of the field. It also changes more centrally and peripherally than pericentrally. These changes are exclusive of any pathological changes (Haas, Flammer, & Schneider, 1986).

Implications for Teaching. Because of the increase in visual changes associated with aging, assessing visual acuity and color perception in older adults is essential before choosing educational materials. Persons with poor vision need materials that have contrasting colors. Pictures should have less detail and figures should be distinctly outlined. Larger print, and more space between figures is also important. Black on white background has been found to be the most readable (Tideiksaar, 1984). Taking non-glossy white paper and black markers into the home for on the spot teaching is helpful if such teaching materials are not available.

Often overlooked is cleanliness of the eye glasses. The older person with poor vision is often unaware of smudges on the lens surface. Hand held magnifying lenses can be used as visual aids that can be brought to the home to illustrate their usefulness. Larger magnifying lenses have less amplification so that the small magnifying glass is a better option. Also, inexpensive reading glasses should not be overlooked when older adults are resistant to having vision tests or corrective lenses.

Each person will have a preferred method of improving his/her vision. It is often better to adapt materials to the older person's usual method than to introduce new visual aids at the same time a client is trying to learn new information or skills (*Ophthalmology*

Update, 1986). When teaching materials cannot be adapted due to the severity of a visual impairment, using audio tapes are an alternative mode for learning (Carter, 1982).

Hearing

Research Findings. Loss of neurons and stiffening of the basilar membrane cause a decreased ability to discriminate speech and increased difficulty in hearing high frequency sounds, particularly soft consonants (e.g., c, ch, f, s, sh, th, and z). Thus, many messages sound garbled and are frequently misunderstood (Corso, 1977; Botwinick, 1984). Hearing loss increases with age. As few as 5 percent are unable to distinguish normal speech at ages 65 to 69. This increases to as many as 30 percent after age 85 (Huntley et al., 1984). The type of hearing deficit makes discrimination of speech from background noises more difficult.

Implications for Teaching. Hearing assessment is important in preparation for teaching. If the person has a hearing aid, verifying that it is on and that the batteries are working is necessary before beginning any other assessment. People without hearing aids, can use head phones commonly used with walkman radios and amplifying devices. An amplifying device with a small radio works by having the radio tuned to a frequency where there is no program. The volume can be turned up or down to change the volume of the voice of the teacher. This allows the learner's and teacher's hands to be free for other tasks. The radios and head sets can be purchased at any store where radio equipment is sold. Many stores have special displays for "assistive hearing devices." Purchase prices are low—usually in the $10 to $30 range. The elderly usually do not resist using these "head sets" since much younger populations use them as well. These same devices can also be used in group settings and are often commonly found in many churches. The portable "assistive hearing devices" are good investments by home care agencies and can be important adjuncts for effective teaching with older groups and individuals (Rupp, Vaughn, & Lightfoot, 1984).

Speaking slightly louder, slower, and in lower tones is helpful in working with the elderly. However, to assure that a message is heard correctly, the individual should repeat back what has been said. Prepared recordings or tapes that can be left with the elderly need to be slower paced (140 words per minute) and in lower tones (Kim, 1981; Hull, 1984). Having head phones plugged into the tape recorder or audio visual teaching material will screen out background noises and enhance discrimination of sound.

Cognitive Changes

Cognitive changes are separated into subsections: (a) intelligence; (b) perception; (c) information processing and cognition; and (d) response time. Although the divisions are somewhat overlapping, separating the components helps to understand the complex cognitive processes. The research findings of each of the four components are discussed first. Because of the difficulty in separating the teaching implications of the four components, they are presented together.

Cognitive Changes and Research Findings

Intelligence. Testing of intelligence is usually not considered under cognitive changes but because of extensive controversy over the differences found in test scores of older and younger adults, a brief discussion is warranted.

Testing intelligence is based on standardized tests that have been designed to forecast academic and professional success for younger populations. Intelligence has been defined as the results of performance on those standardized tests. When educational level was taken into account there were few differences on test results through age sixty. After age 70 test results did decline, but most researchers do not consider the decline to be a valid reflection of the older person's intellectual ability. The standardized tests are inadequate for three reasons: (a) they are designed for the younger person's context, (b) they are usually conducted with elderly who are living in environments very different than those of the younger age group, and (c) they are given without consideration for cohort differences (Willis & Baltes, 1980).

Currently, intelligence tests are not considered of value in determining learning abilities of the older population because they test such a small range of behavior. Additionally, they do not test the range of behavior or knowledge needed by older adults to adapt to their environment. In the research review by Willis & Baltes (1980), the authors suggested that intelligence tests be developed that are age specific and relevant to the life problems and adaptive tasks needed in old age. Because of the limitations of the test measures used, no teaching implications are proposed.

Perception. "Perception" as discussed by Hoyer & Plude (1980), involves time and space dimensions. Time is considered the rapidity that stimuli can be presented for a perception to occur without one stimulus obscuring the next (also referred to as "masking"). In comparing older and younger adults' recall of visual and auditory stimuli, older adults needed more time between the first and second signals for both stimuli to be reported (Welford, 1980; Fozard, 1980; & Hoyer & Plude, 1980). Another pattern called "sequential ordering" was also found to be relevant to the timing of stimuli. In timing between stimuli, younger individuals could integrate the faster paced stimuli more easily, while older adults could integrate the slower presentation of stimuli more easily (Botwinick, 1984; Hoyer &, Plude, 1980). In support of these findings Welford (1980) found that if older subjects were exposed to stimuli for longer periods of time initially, and with a longer time between each exposure, their accuracy of recall was equivalent to younger subjects.

The space dimension of perception refers to the quantity of information that can occupy the attention at any one time (also called parallel processing). The space dimension is tested by presenting subjects with either complex pictures or a number of digits and then asking for immediate recall of as much as can be remembered. Results of the testing showed that up to four digits could be recalled equally well by both young and old. With additional digits, however, recall by young persons exceeded that of older persons (Botwinick, 1984; Welford, 1980). Visual recall of pictures was less conclusive. The elderly did better than younger subjects if the pictures were of familiar content, and there were no distractions during the testing. Younger subjects did better than older adults if conditions were unfamiliar or if there were distractions during the testing. Considerable improvement was obtained with practice by both groups (Botwinick, 1984; Hoyer & Plude, 1980).

Information Processing and Cognition. Cognitive processing includes, memory, problem solving, concept formation, and cognitive training strategies. Each of these components and their research findings are presented.

Memory is commonly divided into short term and long term. For purposes of discussion here, Fozard's (1980) divisions of memory into primary, secondary, and tertiary are used. The three types of memory are defined as follows:

1. primary memory — a short-term store from which information is lost if it is not rehearsed.
2. secondary memory — the store for newly learned information. It is operating when a person is given a set of instructions in order to accomplish a task (also called working memory).
3. tertiary memory — long term memory, or that which can be recalled after long periods of time (e.g., months and years).

The process of remembering is thought to occur in three stages. First primary memory is active for a short period of time, then information moves into secondary memory stores for a longer period and finally moves into tertiary memory for permanent storage.

Experiments have shown that compared to younger age groups, older adults are equally efficient in use of short term memory as long as there are no environmental distractions. After a longer time elapses between the information received and when it is asked to be recalled (when secondary memory must be used), younger age groups excel. However, with training and rehearsal the older groups can approximate younger age groups in secondary memory retrieval (Hartley, Harker, & Walsh, 1980; Fozard, 1980). These experiments have been conducted with information that is new to both younger and older samples. Another factor thought to affect secondary memory of older persons is past experience. It is theorized that older adults are much more discriminating in the use of new information and therefore screen out new information that does not fit with their past experience. Although this may be viewed as a disadvantage, research done by Arenberg (1983) found that linking new material to be learned with information familiar to the older person (e.g., words to places in the house) resulted in recall which equalled that of much younger age groups.

Long term memory (tertiary memory) has been tested by longitudinal studies in which younger and older persons were exposed to the same pictures under laboratory conditions. It was found that there were no differences between younger and older groups in their recall of the pictures two and one half years later (Fozard & Poon, 1976; Kline & Schieber, 1981). For material learned in natural or familiar settings, it has been demonstrated that older adults retained information one to three decades later (Craik, 1977; Schonfield, 1972). Additionally, older adults recalled information specific to their cohort (things that occurred during their life time) better than did younger individuals who learned the same information second hand (Perlmetter, Metzgar, Nezworski, & Miller, 1980).

The tertiary memory has also been tested by asking younger and older subjects for a broad range of information. Older adults were found to have more total knowledge and the efficiency of remembering remained the same across age. In addition, it was noted that older adults were retrieving information from a larger base of stored information than younger adults (Lachman & Lachman, 1980; Botwinick, 1984).

Problems solving and concept formation are not clearly divided. However, problem solving is viewed as a diverse set of procedures. Concept formation is a subset of problem solving in which learning is said to occur by categorization and labeling of objects as belonging or not belonging to a concept. In Giambra & Arenberg's (1980) review of 18 research reports, several approaches to testing age differences in problem solving were noted. Studies that used solving anagram problems, finding embedded figures in pictures, plus a wide range of different problem solving tasks — found no age differences.

In several studies on concept problems, middle age groups (40s and 50s) did better than either the young (18-21) or the older (62-85) groups and that the young made more errors of commission, while the old made more errors of omission (Brinley, Jovick, & McLaughlin, 1974; Falduto & Baron, 1986; Hoyer, Rebok, & Sved, 1979). Other studies, reviewed by Botwinick, (1984) suggested that both problem solving and concept learning were improved when information presented was meaningful to the older adult (Arenberg, 1968, 1974; Reker et al., 1987).

Cognitive training strategies have been used to improve problem solving ability in comparison groups of older and younger adults. In an experiment done by Hartley & Anderson (1986), older adults were asked to guess the location of a square on a checker board by asking the least number of yes and no questions. It was found that older adults could be taught more efficient strategies for using the least number of questions as easily as younger adults. However, age differences were found in continued use of the optimal strategy. Older adults reverted to prior less optimal strategies more often than did younger adults.

Response Time. Slower response time for older adults is the most researched and proven difference between the young and old. Response time is best defined as the time it takes for a person to respond to any stimulus or request. In the past, slowed response time was attributed to slower nerve conduction. However, with more sophisticated testing procedures, slower nerve transmission time cannot be detected. Other central nervous system processes are thought to be responsible (Botwinick, 1984).

Important determinants of a slower response time that have been considered in the elderly include: (a) ability to attend to the task; (b) processing time; and (c) the criterion of confidence.

Attention to the task is more difficult when there are distractions in the situation where testing occurs (e.g., background noise or other events occurring at the same time). Younger adults can better screen out and selectively focus when distractions are present than can older adults (Hoyer & Plude, 1980). Altered perceptions due to deficits in visual or auditory stimuli may also contribute to the increased time it takes to respond to the stimuli (Fozard, 1980; Cunningham, 1980). When messages are clear and presented in an environment free of distraction, response times of older adults compare favorably with response times of the younger age groups (Welford, 1983; Jacewicz & Hartley, 1987).

Processing time is also thought to be increased due to the greater amount of knowledge and experience base against which older adults have to sort and store information. Hartley, Harker, & Walsh compare the slower response time to the computer which decreases its speed of retrieval when there are concurrent demands. He concludes that the person may not have lost processing resources but is simply dealing with higher concurrent processing demands. Another way the increased response time is viewed is that the older adult has to integrate new information with a greater amount of stored knowledge (Botwinick, 1984).

Another explanation for increased response time is called the "criterion of confidence" which is defined as the length of time it takes to answer a question when uncertain of the answer. For the older adult response time was found to be longer than that for a younger person when uncertain of an answer (Welford, 1983; Botwinick, 1984).

Cognitive Changes and Implications for Teaching

The results of experiments related to cognitive changes have been used in intervention research by conducting controlled experiments of learning with older adults. Groups were taught with (a) normally paced methods, (b) slow paced methods, and (c) self paced methods. With normal pacing, younger subjects did better; while with self paced methods learning by the younger and older groups showed very little differences (Ascione & Shimp, 1984; Eisdorfer, Axelrod, & Wilke, 1963; Kim, 1981, 1986).

Differences for older adults in perceptions of time and space dimensions and other learning experiments provide clear evidence for the need to present content more slowly. Older adults need longer exposure to materials with smaller amounts of information in each learning session. More self paced instructional materials are also valuable to aid the learning process (Rendon et al., 1986).

Cognitive processing research demonstrates that the elderly need some adaptations. These include: (a) repeating information in order for secondary memory to function and to increase information storage in long term memory; (b) associating new learning with prior knowledge to improve retention in the secondary memory; and (c) cognitive training that uses meaningful or relevant material for enhancement of problem solving and concept formation. A helpful approach to evaluate processing and cognition and determine if principles being taught are being applied correctly is the "thinking aloud procedure.'' This strategy has been found to enhance learning in older adults. It provides for rehearsal and repetition, and tests the integration and synthesis of knowledge and not just mere recall (Giambra & Arenberg, 1980).

Whatever the cause of slower response time, it is clear that the elderly need to be given more time to respond when presented with new information. Structuring a distraction free environment will help the person to attend to the task. Finding out what is already known will decrease the amount of information that needs to be relayed as well as aid in association of new learning with familiar and relevant information and thereby aid in better retention and less uncertainty.

Motor Dexterity and Mobility

Research Findings

Muscle mass and strength, as well as joint mobility decrease with age. Muscular contraction time and the latency period needed between muscle contractions are prolonged. Decreases in cartilage mass cause a forward flexion of the head and neck, and gentle bending of the elbows, hips and knees. The net effect of these changes is an increase in the amount of energy required to maintain balance and gait (Jacobs, 1981; Rossman, 1979). These effects can be ameliorated with exercise and practice, but age differences will remain. In addition, by age 65, eighty percent of the population have some type of rheumatic complaint (Kane, Kane, & Arnold, 1985).

Difficulty with handling small objects and writing increases from five percent at ages 65-74 to twenty-two percent among persons over 85 (Huntley et al., 1984). The need for assistance with walking also increases with age with only four percent needing help in the 65-74 age group, and forty percent needing help in the over 85 age group (Feller, 1983).

Implications for Teaching

Slower muscle contraction and diminished strength increases the amount of time it takes to perform activities. Additionally, chronic illnesses such as arthritis or past strokes may add to the need for adaptations of learning materials. Teaching methods must be adjusted to the ability and pace of the learner. At times assistive devices are necessary that require consultation with specialists (e.g., physical or occupational therapist). Often, however, the older person has already found ways to adapt to an impairment and can suggest creative ways to adapt procedures to accomplish a task. This can save hours of coordination with other agencies in finding equipment that may be discarded after one or two attempts at use.

Because of individual differences in the amount of joint mobility, it is essential for the client to demonstrate the skills needed to ensure that the required task can be performed. Return demonstrations of skills, even as simple as opening a medication bottle, are important to determine the adjustments needed for the home setting. Teaching of skills (e.g., dressing changes or intravenous medications) will require more time for return demonstrations and practice. Storing items in close proximity to where they will be used is of increased importance when extra energy for movement is required.

Finally, if the client needs help with mobility, the teaching plan should include methods of working out transportation to obtain needed supplies.

A summary of the changes due to aging and their implications for teaching related to sensory, cognitive changes, and motor dexterity are presented in Table 3. Developmental, historical and cohort, and current context influences on learning will be discussed next.

Developmental Tasks of Persons 65 and Over

Research Findings

Developmental tasks are those that result from age changes, along with environmental and cultural factors that are common at certain time periods in the life cycle. Common issues that must be faced by older adults are presented in Table 4. Although in developmental research these tasks are usually grouped together under one age span, they are divided here into 65-74; 75-84; and 85 and over. These groupings will better reflect the changes with age that were previously presented in Table 2.

Life and interests in the early retirement years are quite different than those after 85. For example, in early retirement most of the

TABLE 3. Teaching Implications for Common Differences in Older Adults

Cognitive Changes	Affect on Learning	Teaching Implications
Slower nerve transmission	Slowed reception time Slowed reaction time Increase in amount of time for learning	Use materials that permit client to control the pace of lerning. Speech and tapes @140 words per minute. Wait and check understanding before changing topics.
Decreased short term memory	May forget what is new material	Need repeated segments Senses activated (repeat, in writing, visuals)
Increased background of already learned information that must be integrated	Will not easily accept new information that is not congruent with what already "know" Easier to overload with sensory input	Find out what already doing related to material to be taught. Clear up misconceptions. Add only what necessary. connect with what already believe. Less material presented in each learning segment Keep sentences short

Visual Changes

Decreased acuity	Minimize detail in illustrations
	Use large print and double space
Decreased accomodation	Use highly contrasting colors (black on yellow is best contrast for most people)
Decreased lens transparency	Light sources should be bright without producing a glare
Decreased ability to distinguish details	Make sure learner's glasses are clean
Reduced ability to see in dim light	Provide magnifying aids
Decreased ability to distinguish colors	
May not know glasses are not clean	

Hearing Changes

Decreased perception of high frequencies	Have learner repeat back what was heard
	Use tapes with head phones and carefully chosen words
Decreased ability to screen out other noise	Eliminate background noise such as radio or T.V.
Harder to hear c, ch, f, s, sh, t, z	Use audio aids when teaching
Background noise will decrease what is heard	Use more visual illustrations

Motor Dexterity

Slowed nerve transmission	Allow adequate time for return demonstrations
May have arthritic changes or tremors	Make certain can perform procedures required and help with adaptations. Use consultants for adaptive equipment. Place things within easy reach and in areas used by learner.
Cannot move as quickly	
Difficulty with hard movements of ambulation	

TABLE 4. Developmental Tasks for Persons over Sixty-five

CENTRAL PROCESSES: Accepting the shifting of generational roles
Mutual Aid versus Uselessness
Ego Integrity versus Despair

Ages 65-74
Retirement

1. Adjust living standards to retirement income and supplement with remunerative activity as able.
2. Pursue new interests and maintain former activities to gain sense of being needed.
3. Decision making regarding care giving role for friends and relatives.
4. For women - adjust to death of spouse.
5. For men - continue close supportive relationship with spouse.
6. Maintain interest in people outside family and in social, civic and political interests.

Ages 75-84

Adjusting
to chronic
illness.

Meaningful
integration.

1. Deciding where and how to live out remaining years.
2. Find a satisfactory living arrangement and work out safe, comfortable household routine.
3. Maintain contact with children, grandchildren and other relatives and find emotional satisfaction with them.
4. Support younger generation in their more central role.
5. Maintain maximum level of health care and health practices.
6. Men - adjust to loss of spouse.

Ages 85 +

Living in face
of death.

Self-acceptance.

1. Find meaning in life in face of decreasing energy and loss of significant others.
2. Find and adjust to more protective living environments as necessary.
3. Recognize own dependency needs and be able to accept assistance when needed.
4. Develop relationships with younger generations.
5. Engage in life review and transmission of family and cultural history to younger generations.
6. Maintain sense of self-esteem (usefulness) in the face of societal stereotypes and declining health or strength.

These tasks are an integration of: Carter & McGoldrick's (1980) "Stages of Family Life Cycle"; Duvall's (1977) "Eight Stages of Family Life", (1977); Erikson's (1963) "Psychosocial Development"; Murray & Zentner's (1979) "Developmental Tasks"; and Rhodes' (1977) "Life Cyle";

elderly still have a spouse to help provide health care while after 85, it is more likely that the younger generation will be needed to offer assistance. Also, by 85 diminishing abilities may have necessitated several changes in living situations as well as a greater need for dependence on others for basic needs. The developmental issues outlined in Table 4 will determine what teaching adaptations are needed.

Teaching Implications and Developmental Considerations

Being aware of common developmental issues during different age groups of older adults leads to awareness of how to adapt teaching to income levels, fitting new learning into going chronic illness regimens, and evaluating whether losses that are occurring are interfering with the person's ability to learn. Role shifts due to losses or increasing dependency can be of much greater concern than learning new information. Helping the client to negotiate assistance from relatives or friends in order to regain health or maintain a degree of independence may take priority over teaching other information. Teaching sessions can include family members who will be involved in supporting an elderly couple, and may consequently save the teacher many hours of wasted instruction time.

Historical and Cohort Influences

Historical factors unique to the aged include cohort effects and each individual's own life experience. Cohort effects are those common experiences and influences that occur as a result of being born at a particular time. Thus persons born in the early 1900s will have quite a different set of influences that form a basis for their beliefs, attitudes and actions than will those persons born in the 1940s.

Research Findings

Cohort effects common to those who were born in 1920 and 1930 are such factors as less educational opportunity, living through the Depression, and the experience of World War II. Of persons born in 1900, fifty percent have only a fifth grade education, while those born in the 1920s, fifty percent have an 8th grade education (Birren, Munnichs, Thomae, & Marois, 1983). Current educational levels of persons in older age groups have been presented in Table 2.

Persons who lived through the 1930s as adults are often much less willing to spend as much on health care than those born in the 1940s or 1950s. Of men born in the late 20s and early 30s (now 60-65 years of age) three out of four are veterans (Veteran's Administration, 1985). Veteran funds can, therefore, be a reimbursement source for health care for men in this age group.

Besides cohort influences, consideration of personal and cultural background is important. Older individuals have learned much through their experiences. As a result they are much less likely to accept new information without considering how it fits with what they believe already works for them. In health matters in particular, the elderly have often developed habits for staying healthy or dealing with symptoms. Suggestions or teaching especially from younger persons, is often not accepted without checking with their age peers as to its value (Ebersole & Hess, 1985).

Implications for Teaching

Because of the wide differences in personal experience, assessment of what the client and family already know and are doing related to the planned teaching becomes essential prior to offering advice. It is important to ask about the client's knowledge as well as what may have been learned from other people with the same illness or treatment regimen. Once a common baseline of information is established, the home care professional can decide with the client the most important learning needs (Doak, Doak, & Root, 1985).

Second in importance is knowledge of the educational background and literacy level prior to preparing and selecting learning materials. It is important to recognize that years of education frequently do not translate into literacy levels (Doak et al.) One test of reading materials suggested by several sources (Doak et al.; McLaughlin, 1969; Smith, 1987c) is the SMOG grading system for educational materials. This system involves counting the number of syllables in words in selected sections of teaching materials. Having the person read several short paragraphs of the standard teaching materials and then explain in his or her own words what it means is helpful in determining if those materials are understood. Use of more easily understood vocabulary is helpful not only in adapting written materials, but in selecting vocabulary to use for verbal instruction. Visual aids can also be used that provide pictorial representations rather than word reminders. These pictures often need to be invented with the help of the learner so that meanings and reminders are clear (Doak, et al.; Dunn et al., 1985). The SMOG grading system, and a pictorial example for persons with low literacy skills are found in Appendix B.

Current Contexts of Older Adults

The last area to be considered is the current environment and situation in which the aged person lives. Within the current context, usual daily routines, key psychosocial and health stressors, social support, and environmental resources are all important for timing and tailoring the teaching to the situation.

Research Findings

Research findings indicate that people prefer information about and help in fitting medications or treatments into their daily life, rather than information about actions of drugs or the reasons treatments are needed (Ascione & Shimp, 1984). Health behavior of the elderly has been shown to be markedly improved by giving priority to helping the elderly adopt alternative ways to meet medication and treatment needs. This has been proved to be even more effective than offering information about disease symptoms, medication side effects or treatment regimens.

Psychosocial factors that need attention have been reviewed under developmental issues. They will, however, appear in different configurations for each individual. Health stressors may be insidious or sudden in onset, slowly progressive or punctuated by remissions and exacerbations. Management of the illness may require few changes in routines, or may be complex and require major changes in the daily life style and living situation. Medications are a major consideration in timing of teaching. They can either diminish or increase a person's ability to pay attention to information that is presented or to do required tasks (Strauss et al., 1984).

In the early stages of an illness or for acute episodes, family and neighbors may be a major source of support. However, research reports have shown that if illness is prolonged (as is the case with many chronic diseases of the elderly), social supports tend to diminish over time (Strauss et al., 1984; Litwak, 1985; Antonnucci, 1985). Formal supports, such as doctors and agencies, may be available but poorly coordinated. As noted earlier, monetary resources diminish with age and so may not be available for acquiring formal services. The presence or absence of stairs, qualities of the neighborhood, and protectiveness of the living environment will determine how much self care can be expected.

Implications for Teaching

Each area of the older person's current context: (a) daily routines; (b) psychosocial and health stressors; (c) social supports; and (d) environmental resources need to be evaluated for teaching to be integrated with the person's abilities and resources.

Daily Routines. The expected medication regimen, personal care, or new procedure being taught may make daily life much more complicated for the individual. Difficulties posed in acquiring needed supplies, or disagreement between family members about the importance of health behaviors all need attention. By asking about expected difficulties, adjustments can be made and the learner can become an effective participant in the planning and implementation of the teaching plan.

Psychosocial and Health Stressors. The major emphasis in assessing psychosocial and health stressors, concerns how stressors affect the ability to concentrate, remember, and solve problems. The best timing for teaching can be planned for those periods during the day when the person feels the best or likes to read or do something active. For example, the best time for learning may be at peak effect of their medication or may be before the side effects of a medication have caused drowsiness or blurred vision.

Asking what things are going on now that are causing stress or worry will be helpful in ascertaining the client's stress level. In addition, asking about recent positive events will aid in discovering sources of motivation and pleasure. This information will be helpful in encouraging health behaviors that decrease stress or increase pleasurable experiences. Motivation for learning is greater when factors that facilitate or inhibit the client's ability to learn are recognized by the teacher. After essential information has been relayed and demonstrated, and the learner has had a chance to practice with supervision, the teacher needs to continue to ask the client for explicit feedback and concerns to adapt teaching to changes that arise.

Social Supports. It is important to obtain information about people who can help the client when physical or emotional problems occur. Asking the client who else should be taught new information in case of an emergency, is a helpful approach. The distance supportive individuals live from the client is an important factor in judging availability of a friend or relative. Litwak (1985) found that if helpers were more than twenty minutes away, it was rare that assistance was provided.

Environmental Resources. Income is important to determine if purchasing medical equipment, making adaptations in the home, or buying educational materials requires money over and above the client's insurance reimbursements. Asking if there is difficulty in meeting monthly expenses has been found to be more helpful than knowing the exact income of the client. Any effect financial problems might have on applying new information can then be discussed with the client.

Summary

It becomes apparent through the literature review that older adults need teaching adapted to their special needs or circumstances. The high degree of variability among the aged, their sensory, cognitive, mobility, developmental, historical, and current circumstances all need to be taken into account in order for cognitive, psychomotor, and affective learning to occur. The wide variability in the learning abilities of older adults requires an assessment to determine what necessary adaptations are before an effective plan can be developed. A suggested assessment guide that incorporates the previous discussion is provided in Appendix C. The information in the assessment guide may already be available through the usual physical or social assessments conducted by agency personnel. If so, the guide can be used to review the record and note the areas of strengths and deficits before establishing a teaching plan and collecting teaching resources. Because client teaching is reimburseable through Medicare and insurance, a documented assessment can be an important means for acquiring the funds necessary for teaching time.

IMPORTANT GUIDELINES FOR TEACHING THE ELDERLY

Four basic questions should be addressed to develop teaching plans: (a) what is the purpose of teaching? (b) who should be taught? (c) what should be taught, and (d) how should it be taught?

The first question provides direction for the teacher's actions. The second question requires decisions as to whether the material should be taught at the community level, in small groups, to family members, to the ill person, or to various combinations of those just named. The third question requires determining what information is important to be taught. The final question requires evaluating readiness and constructing the teaching plan utilizing the cognitive, affective, and psychomotor domains.

Purpose

The purpose of teaching the elderly is not different from that of any other age group. The central purpose is to enable individuals and families to deal effectively with their responses to health issues and illness. This purpose is accomplished through:

a. Providing information to clients about illness management and health promotion;
b. Helping clients and their families learn new skills and increase their ability for self-care; and
c. Assisting clients and their families in adapting to changes in lifestyle brought on by illness or aging (Loustau, 1986).

Who to Teach

To gain the most from teaching, it is important to spend time in staff conferences determining the teaching needs common to a segment of clients that could be taught effectively in community wide or small group settings. Health promotion and general medication taking advice is often best delivered in a community wide effort, through public television at times when most older adults watch. Small support groups are often helpful for learning about specific chronic illness management regimens because individuals can share alternative ways for accomplishing the same objectives (Pesznecker & Zahlis, 1986). Support groups for the elderly who are dealing with caregiving issues or loss of loved ones are two of the most common resources types of support groups. If such alternatives are not available, the home health agency can be instrumental in developing such groups or promoting their development through other community programs. Family caregivers of ill elders gain much needed information and support from each other in such groups. (Appendix D provides a list of helpful resources for developing support groups.)

Specific procedures or treatments that individuals must adapt necessitates in-home teaching and requires planning to determine what family or neighbor support persons should be present for teaching sessions. Discussion at agency staff meetings concerning mechanisms for getting the client's family members to come to in-home teaching sessions can improve the use of teaching time.

What to Teach

Although each individual has some unique learning needs, there is common developmental and physical health information that can enhance the health of older adults. The basic needs of nutrition, exercise, rest, and social activities, and the importance of routine health check ups are some of the most obvious areas of relevance. A recent article by Kane, Kane, and Arnold (1986) reviews areas of important teaching for older adults and lists the following areas as necessary for them to be informed health care consumers and to reduce their risks of accidents or poor health:

Preventive activities for heart disease, stroke, cancer, broken hips, and infectious diseases such as influenza, pneumonia, and tuberculosis.

Behaviors likely to produce beneficial or adverse effects on health status. These include smoking, diet modification, exercise, weight control, social participation and stress reduction.

Problems requiring attention for health providers. These include visual and hearing impairment, dentition, foot problems, depression, alcohol abuse, and urinary incontinence.

Iatrogenic problems are those that result from the health care providers. The most common are adverse drug reactions or side effects. Others include nosocomial infections and functional disability created by overprotective environments. (pp. 951-952)

Kane's article gives an excellent overview of important health information for elders and detailed information of what is important to teach in each of the areas listed above. The article also discusses research studies that demonstrate education campaigns resulting in better self care by older community members as measured by such factors as (a) fewer visits to physicians due to adverse drug reactions, and (b) more cancers being detected in earlier and treatable stages.

Group settings are often best for teaching about developmental needs of the elderly. Content areas to include are changing roles and relationships in older families; health issues associated with aging; available community resources; how to deal with stresses of giving care to older family members; legal issues for older adults and their families; and choosing appropriate living arrangements (resources for developing groups on these topics are provided in Appendix D).

How to Teach

The teacher in the home care setting must realize that teaching is not simply advising or relaying information. It is based on a collaborative relationship with the client that is established during the assessment and planning phase of the teaching-learning process and is continuous through the intervention and evaluation phases. Determining readiness for learning and determining the appropriate approach, requires attention to cognitive, affective, and psychomotor domains which are all important for effective learning.

Determining Readiness and Establishing Rapport

Learning readiness can be evaluated by listening to the client's questions and concerns. If the client does not volunteer questions, then asking the client about major concerns or worries can help in evaluating whether there are stressors that will interfere with learning new information. Listening to the learner's concerns sympathetically and asking what would be helpful to them in addressing those concerns is the most valuable first step in establishing rapport and in determining priorities in teaching. Acknowledging or attending to the client's priorities first will increase the learner's readiness for involvement in the learning process (Smith, 1986c). Readiness is usually apparent when the client asks questions about the illness and asks what can be done about problems that need attention.

In determining readiness and assessing how to teach, cognitive, affective, and psychomotor domains of the teaching-learning process all need to be considered. The learner may have all the necessary knowledge and skill to manage an illness, but may have feelings that prevent the actual performance of those behaviors. Within each phase of the teaching plan (assessment, planning, interventions, and evaluation) identifying which domains to address is a joint venture of the teacher and learner.

The Cognitive Domain

Cognitive assessment includes finding out what the client's knowledge is about the information to be learned. Asking questions regarding what is known about a procedure or disease or what knowledge has been gained from other people is part of the cognitive assessment. Asking what the learner wants to know aids in joint planning about what to teach. Too much information or irrelevant information can be circumvented by accurate assessment of the knowledge base. This determination focuses on teaching only the most essential information. A short pretest can often stimulate discussion as well as determine what points need most attention.

Cognitive interventions and evaluation include verbal, visual, and demonstration modes of instruction. The materials and methods can be adapted to the learner by basing the information on the prior cognitive assessment.

Evaluation of what has been learned can be gained through asking the learner to write an explanation of important points, or demonstrate a procedure or skill (Smith, 1987b).

The Affective Domain

Affective assessment and planning is acquired by asking the person about fears, feelings, beliefs, and concerns they have about disease or procedure. It also includes asking about family or friends and their beliefs or attitudes about what is to be taught. Cooperation with family and friends is important in developing a teaching plan. The attitudes and actions of the elderly are often affected by family or friends who assist them (King, 1984).

Motivation for learning the procedure can be assessed through noting the learner's responsiveness during the assessment. A client's inattention to instruction or hesitancy in sharing information is usually a sign that the client is not ready to learn and signifies that other problems may need further exploration.

Affective interventions require the teacher to be responsive to the learner's concerns by reaching agreements on the learner's beliefs and attitudes, and by allowing the learner to discuss feelings and concerns. Better outcomes can be obtained by adapting health regimens to the life style and concerns of the learner. Evaluating the affective domain requires observing whether the learner listens and asks questions, reports important information or problems, and follows through consistently with the agreed on plans. When behavior does not reflect that affective learning has occurred, the teacher and learner's desired outcomes may be in conflict and need further discussion and planning (Smith, 1987b).

The Psychomotor Domain

Psychomotor assessment and planning includes not only whether the client has the physical and mental capacity to perform a procedure or comply with a health regimen, but whether the environment and resources are supportive to accomplishing the task. Asking about the availability of money or transportation to acquire supplies or discussing neighborhood safety to permit a prescribed amount of walking are examples of psychomotor assessment. These areas are often overlooked in planning with the client. As discussed earlier, any psychomotor assessment involving performance necessitates observing the client actually doing the task.

The psychomotor domain interventions require demonstration of procedures or skills, enlisting the learner's help in timing teaching sessions, and adapting the skill or procedure to the learner's environment. Evaluation of psychomotor activities are through direct observation or the clients report (Smith, 1987b). Modification can be made and help from the client's family and friends enlisted when the client is unable to perform activities independently.

In summary, attention to the learner's readiness and to each of the three domains of learning need to be included in the teaching-learning process. Basing the teaching on the assessment, enhances the likelihood that content will be limited to what is most important to the client, and that those who need to be involved in the learning process will be enlisted. Thus, the manner in which information is relayed and incorporated into the life of the learner will more likely produce the outcomes that have been jointly agreed on by the teacher and learner (see Table 5 for an overview of important points on how to teach).

CONCLUSION

In the teaching and learning process, assessment, planning, intervention and evaluation does not occur at one point in time. They are an ongoing process. This paper has provided an overview of the teaching and learning process with special attention given to research results and their implications for the older adult. Tables have summarized important points and the appendixes contain suggestions for additional resources. In addition to the appendixes referred to in the paper, there is a learner assessment guide and a mental status examination that has been found by the author to be especially helpful as a screening tool for cognitive impairment (see Appendix C). Appendix D provides resources that can be obtained for

TABLE 5. Important Guidelines for Determining How to Teach

A. Readiness and Rapport

* Enhance readiness for learning by providing assistance with issues that are most important to the client.

* Establish rapport by listening to the learner's concerns and planning with them for learning activities.

B. Cognitive Domain

* Find out what the client already knows or has learned from others about information or skills that need to be taught. Find out what the client wants to know.

* Relate new learning to past knowledge and learning.

* Teach only what is essential and what is requested. Choose instruction methods that allow for self-pacing of learning and opportunities for rehearsal and feedback.

B. Affective Domain

* Determine what attitudes and beliefs the learner has about their illness or health regimen.

* Collaborate with the learner regarding the best methods of adapting new learning to their life style.

* Plan for inclusion of family and support person's in teaching sessions.

* Establish desirable outcomes in collaboration with the client and or family that enhance motivation and self-care.

C. Psychomotor Domain

* Assess strengths and needs for adapting teaching methods with special attention to vision, hearing, and cognitive abilities.

* Be alert for aiding the family or client in selecting a more protective environment for health or illness care to safeguard family integrity or client's health.

* Provide clear methods of continuity and access to health agencies for answering important questions that may arise in absence of the teacher.

the library of a home health agency for use in developing teaching plans, programs for groups, and educational materials for clients and families.

Throughout the paper the importance of tailoring the teaching to the learner's needs and abilities has been stressed. Because of the unique needs of older adults and the importance of not overloading the learner with unnecessary information, assessment is the most crucial phase of the teaching-learning process. Determination of learning needs can be integrated into the usual assessments that are required of home care staff. Time and effort are reduced by initially determining readiness and planning with the client for desired outcomes. Becoming more aware of whether the client concerns are cognitive, affective, and/or psychomotor helps focus teaching, and serves as a basis for documenting important teaching modalities. When teaching is tailored to the learner, the client feels more able to incorporate learning and attain the degree of independence needed for remaining in the home setting.

REFERENCES

Antonnucci, T. (1985). Personal characteristics, social support and social behavior. In R. Binstock & E. Shanas (Eds.). *Handbook of aging and the social sciences* (2nd ed.). New York: Van Nostrand Reinhold.

Arenberg, D. (1968). Concept problem solving in young and old adults. *Journal of Gerontology, 23,* 279-282.

Arenberg, D. (1974). A longitudinal study of problem solving in adults. *Journal of Gerontology, 29,* 650-658.

Arenberg, D. (1983). Memory and learning do decline later in life. In J. Birren, J. Munnichs, H. Thomae, & M. Marois. *Aging: A challenge to science and society.* (pp. 312-322). New York: Oxford University Press.

Ascione, F.J., & Shimp, L.S. (1984). The effectiveness of four education strategies in the elderly. *Drug Intelligence and Clinical Pharmacology, 18,* 1-12.

Birren, J., Munnichs, J., Thomae, H., & Marois, M. (1983). *Aging: A challenge to science and society (vl 3).* New York: Oxford University Press.

Bloom, B., Englehart, M., Furst, E., Hill, W., & Krathwohl, D. (1956). *Taxonomy of educational objectives, Handbook I: Cognitive domain.* New York: David McKay Company, Inc.

Botwinick, J. (1984). *Aging and behavior: A comprehensive integration of research findings.* New York: Springer Publishing Company.

Brinley, F., Jovick, T., & McLaughlin, L. (1974). Age, reasoning and memory in adults. *Journal of Gerontology, 29,* 182-189.

Carnevali, D., & Patrick, M. (1986). *Nursing management for the elderly.* (2nd edition). New York: Lippincott.

Carter, E., & McGoldrick, M. (Eds.) (1980). *The family life cycle: A framework for family therapy.* New York: Gardner Press.

Carter, P.D. (1982). Sensory changes with age: Implications for learning and research. *Lifelong Learning* (June), 19-21.

Corso, J. (1977). Auditory perception and communication. In J. Birren, & K. Schaie (Eds.). *Handbook of psychology of aging.* New York: Von Nostrand Reinhold, pp. 535-553.

Craik, F. (1977). Age differences in long term memory. In J. Birren, & W. Schaie (Eds.). *Handbook of psychology of aging.* New York: Von Nostrand Reinhold.

Cunningham, W. (1980). Speed, age, and qualitative differences in cognitive functioning. In L.W. Poon (Ed.). *Aging in the 1980s.* Washington D.C.: American Psychological Association.

Doak, C., Doak, L., & Root, J. (1985). *Teaching patients with low literacy skills.* Philadelphia: J.P. Lippincott Co.

Dunn, M.M., Buckwalter, K.C., Weinstein, L.B., & Palti, H. (1985). Innovations in family and community health: Teaching the illiterate client does not have to be a problem. *Family and Community Health, 8* (3), 76-80.

Duvall, E. (1977). *Family development* (5th ed.). Philadelphia: W.B. Lippincott Company.

Ebersole, P., & Hess, P. (1985). *Toward healthy aging: Human needs and nursing response.* St. Louis: The C.V. Mosby Company.

Eisdorfer, C., Axelrod, S., & Wilke, F. (1963). Stimulus exposure and time as a factor in serial learning in an aged sample. *Journal of Abnormal Psychology, 67,* 594 +

Erikson, E.H. (1963). *Childhood and society* (2nd. ed.). New York: Norton.

Falduto, L., & Baron, A. (1986). Age-related effects of practice and task complexity on card sorting. *Journal of Gerontology, 41,* 659-661.

Feller, B.A. (1983). Americans needing help to function at home. *NCHS Advancedata, 92,* (Sept. 14). DSHS Publication No. (PHS) 83-1250.

Folstein, M.F., Folstein, S., & McHugh, P.R. (1975). Mini-mental state: A practical method for grading the cognitive state of patients for the clinician. *Journal of Psychiatric Research, 12,* 189-198.

Fozard, J. (1980). The time for remembering. In L.W. Poon (Ed.). *Aging in the 1980s.* Washington D.C.: American Psychological Association.

Fozard, J., & Poon, L. (1976). *Effects of age on long term retention of pictures.* Technical report 76-02, Boston: GRECC, Veterans Administration.

Giambra, L., & Arenberg, D. (1980). Problem solving, concept learning, and aging. In L.W. Poon (Ed.). *Aging in the 1980s.* Washington D.C.: American Psychological Association.

Haas, A., Flammer, J., & Schneider, V. (1986). Influence of age on the visual fields of normal subjects. *American Journal of Ophthalmology 101,* 199-223.

Hallburg, J.C. (1976). The teaching of aged adults. *Journal of Gerontological Nursing, 2* (3), 13-19.

Hartley, A., & Anderson, J. (1986). Instruction, induction, generation, and evaluation of strategies for solving search problems. *Journal of Gerontology, 41*, 650-658.

Hartley, J., Harker, J., & Walsh, D. (1980). Contemporary issues and new directions in adult development of learning and memory. In L.W. Poon (Ed.). *Aging in the 1980s.* Washington D.C.: American Psychological Association.

Horn, B.(Principal Investigator), (1986). *Elderly homecare project.* (Unpublished preliminary report). Funded by Fred Meyer Charitable Trust. Seattle, WA: University of Washington, School of Nursing, Community Health Care Systems.

Hoyer, W, & Plude, D. (1980). Attentional and perceptual processes in the study of cognitive aging. In L.W. Poon (Ed.). *Aging in the 1980s.* Washington D.C.: American Psychological Association.

Hoyer, W., Rebok, G., & Sved, S. (1979). Effects of varying irrelevant information on adult age differences in problem solving. *Journal of Gerontology, 34*, 553-560.

Hull, R. (1984). Talking to the hearing impaired older person. In J. Birren, J. Munnichs, H. Thomae, & M. Marois. *Aging: A challenge to science and society.* (p. 194). New York: Oxford University Press.

Huntley, J., Brock, D., Ostfeld, A., Taylor, J., & Wallace, R. (1984). *Established populations for epidemiologic studies of the elderly.* National Institute on Aging: USDHHS, NIH Publication No. 86-2443.

Jacewicz, M., & Hartley, A., (1987). Age differences in the speed of cognitive operations: Resolution of inconsistent findings. *Journal of Gerontology, 42*, 86-88.

Jacobs, R. (1981). Physical changes in the aged. In M. Devereaux (Ed.). *Elder care: A guide to clinical geriatrics.* New York: Grune & Stratton, Inc.

Kane, R.L., Kane, R.A., & Arnold, S.B. (1985). Prevention and the elderly: Risk factors. *Health Services Research, 19,* (6, Part II), 945-1005.

Kim, K. (1986). Response time and health care learning of elderly clients. *Research in Nursing and Health, 9,* 233-239.

Kim, K.K., & Grier, M.R. (1981). Pacing effects of medication instruction for the elderly. *Journal of Gerontological Nursing, 7* (8), 464-468.

King, E. (1984). *Affective education in nursing.* Rockville, MD: Apsen.

Kleoppel, J., & Henry, D. (1987). Teaching patients, families, and communities about their medications. In C. Smith (Ed). *Patient education: Nurses in partnership with other health professionals.* Orlando, FL: Grune & Stratton, Inc. pp. 293-295.

Kline, D., & Schieber, F. (1981). What are the age differences in visual sensory memory? *Journal of Gerontology, 36,* 86-89.

Krathwohl, D., Bloom, B., & Masia, B. (1964).*Taxonomy of educational objectives, Handbook II: Affective domain.* New York: David McKay Company, Inc.

Lachman, J., & Lachman, R. (1980). Age and the actualization of world knowledge. In L. Poon, J. Fozard, L. Cermak, D. Arenberg, & L.W. Thompson (Eds.). *New directions in memory and aging* (Chapter 18 pp. 285-311). Hillsdale, NJ: Lawrence Erlbaum Associates.

Litwak, E. (1985). *Helping the elderly.* New York: Guilford Press.

Loustau, A. (1986). Health promotion and patient teaching. In M. Patrick, S. Woods, R. Craven, J. Rokosky, & P. Bruno. *Medical surgical nursing: Pathophysiological concepts* (pp. 42-48). New York: J.P. Lippincott.

Manton, K., Siegler, & Woodbury, M. (1986). Patterns of intellectual development in later life. *Journal of Gerontology, 41,* 486-499.

McLaughlin, G.H. (1969). SMOG grading—a new readability formula. *Journal of Reading,* (May), 639-646.

Murray, R., & Zentner, J.P. (1979). *Nursing assessment & health promotion throughout the life span.* (2nd edition). Englewood Cliffs, NJ: Prentice-Hall, Inc.

_____ Ophthalmology Update (1986). Presentation at Fifth National Conference for Nurse Practitioners (Oct 1st): Sante Fe, NM.

Pelmutter, M., Metzger, R., Nezworski, T., & Miller, K. (1981). Spatial and temporal memory in 20 and 60 year olds. *Journal of Gerontology, 36,* 59-65.

Pesznecker, B., Horn, B., Werner, J., & Kenyon, V. (1987). Home health services in a climate of cost containment. *Home Health Services Quarterly, 8,* (1), 5-21.

Pesznecker, B., & Zahlis, E. (1986). Establishing mutual-help groups for the family-member care givers: A new role for community health nurses. *Public Health Nursing, 3* (1), 29-37.

Redman, B., (1984). *The process of patient education* (5th edition). St. Louis: C.V. Mosby Company.

Reilly, D. (1980). *Behavioral objectives—evaluation in nursing* (2nd ed.). New York: Appleton-Century-Crofts.

Reker, G., Peacock, E., & Wong, P. (1987). Meaning and purpose in late life and well-being: A life-span perspective. *Journal of Gerontology, 42,* 44-49.

Rendon, D., Davis, K., Gioliella, E., & Tranzillo, M. (1986). The right to know the right to be taught. *Journal of Gerontological Nursing, 12,* 33-38.

Rhodes, S. (1977). A developmental approach to the life cycle of the family. *Social Casework, 58,* 301-311.

Rossman, I. (1979). Anatomy of aging. In I. Rossman (ed.). *Clinical geriatrics* (2nd edition). Philadelphia: J.P. Lippincott.

Rupp, R., Vaughn, G., & Lightfoot, R. (1984). Nontraditional 'aids' to hearing: Assistive listening devices. *Geriatrics, 39,* (3), 55-73.

Schonfield, D. (1972). Theoretical nuances and practical old questions: The psychology of Aging. *Canadian Psychologist, 13,* 262-266.

Simpson, E. (1972). *The classification of educational objectives in the psychomotor domain* Vol. 3, Mt. Rainer, MD: Gryphon House, Inc.

Smith, C.E. (1987a). Nurses' increasing responsibility for patient education. In

C.E. Smith, (Ed.). *Patient education: Nurses in partnership with other professionals* (pp. 3-30). New York: Grune & Stratton, Inc.

Smith, C.E. (Ed.) (1987b). *Patient education: Nurses in partnership with other professionals.* New York: Grune & Stratton, Inc.

Smith, C.E. (1987c). Using the teaching process to determine what to teach and how to evaluate learning. In C.E. Smith, (Ed.). *Patient education: Nurses in partnership with other professionals* (pp. 61-96). New York: Grune & Stratton, Inc.

Spar, J.E. (1982). Dementia in the aged. *Psychiatric Clinics of North America, 5,* 65087.

Strauss, A., Corbin, J., Faberhaugh, S., Glaser, B., Maines, D., Suczek, B., & Wiener, C. (1984). *Chronic illness and the quality of life* (2nd ed.). St. Louis: C.V. Mosby Co.

Tideiksaar, R. (1984). Guidelines for teaching the adult learner. *Physicians Assistant,* (Dec), 46-53.

U.S. Department of Commerce (1985). *Statistical abstracts of the United States* (105th ed.). Washington, D.C.: U.S. Govt. Printing Office.

Veterans Administration (1985). *Annual Report 1985.* Washington, D.C. Office of Administrator of Veterans Affairs.

Welford, A. (1980). Relationships between reaction time and fatigue, stress, age and sex. In A. Welford (Ed,), *Reaction times* (pp. 321-354). New York: Academic Press.

Welford, A. (1983). Perception, memory and motor performance. In J. Birren, J. Munnichs, H. Thomae, & M. Marois. *Aging: A challenge to science and society.* (pp. 297-311). New York: Oxford University Press.

Willis, S., & Baltes, P. (1980). Intelligence in adulthood and aging: Contemporary issues. In L.W. Poon (Ed.). *Aging in the 1980s.* Washington D.C.: American Psychological Association.

APPENDIX A

TERMINOLOGY FOR WRITING BEHAVIORAL OBJECTIVES

I. COGNITIVE DOMAIN

   A. Level 1 Knowledge and comprehension
      (defines, identifies, lists, names, recalls, states
      recognize, gives examples, reports, summarizes)

   B. Level 2 Application and analysis
      (changes, modifies, prepares, shows, uses
      illustrates, compares, selects)

   C. Level 3 Synthesis and Evaluation
      (explains, organizes, classifies, plans, justifies, assesses)

II. AFFECTIVE DOMAIN

   A. Level 1 Receiving
      (asks, chooses, describes, follows)

   B. Level 2 Responding
      (answers, assists, complies, discusses, reads, reports, writes)

   C. Level 3 Valuing
      (accepts, acts, completes, shares, helps, performs, assumes, is consistent,
      questions, defends)

III. PSYCHOMOTOR DOMAIN

    A.

        Level 1 Perception and Set
              (chooses, selects, separates, responds starts, volunteers)

    B.

        Level 2 Guided Response
              (demonstrates, fastens, fixes, manipulates, measures)

    C.

        Level 3 Adaptation and Organization
              (adapts, changes, revises, arranges, creates, designs)

The terminology has been selected from Bloom et al., 1956; Krathwohl et al., 1964; and Simpson, 1972.

TEACHING AND LEARNING ASSESSMENT GUIDE FOR OLDER ADULTS

Areas of Assessment	Method of Assessment	Planned Adaptations in Learning Materials
A. **Readiness for Learning**	Ask for major concerns	Use this column to record results and ways to adapt teaching materials
B. **Cognitive Assessment**		
Learner's knowledge	Ask what already know about subject Determine reading level	
Literacy Level	Ask for educational level and have person read a portion of usual educational materials (Use SMOG test to assess materials)	
Memory & Thinking	Mini-Mental State Exam (MMS) Notice pace of responses during MMS	
C. **Affective Learning**		
Motivation	Find out what they are most concerned about and what think most need to know and adapt incentives for learning to those concerns	

Environment and Situation

Monthly income, or ask if can afford to buy any needed equipment or supplies. Ask what is being spent monthly on medications

Ask about transportation to obtain supplies, and driving ability. If cannot obtain own supplies who does and how available are they.

Recent, current, and future sources of stress

Any recent deaths or losses of family or friends

Recent changes of residence

Key Sources of Support

Ask learner who else should learn what being taught in case unable to do own care. Get names addresses and phone numbers.

Obtain list of physicians or other agencies being used to coordinate teaching effort

D. Psychomotor Assessment

Hearing

Whisper test

Presence of hearing aid

Which is best ear for hearing

Notice during MMS if repeating back words correctly

Vision

Notice if wears glasses and be sure they are clean before testing vision.

Use small Roserbaum chart or various sizes of news print to determine print size for educational materials.

Ask if difficulty distinguishing colors

Motor Dexterity and Mobility

Observe hand movements for dexterity, tremors and strengths

APPENDIX B

THE SMOG GRADING SCALE FOR EDUCATIONAL MATERIALS

READABILITY TESTING

1. Count 10 consecutive sentences near the beginning, in the middle, and near the end of the text.

2. Circle all of the words containing three or more syllables (polysyllabic), including repetitions of the same word.

3. Total the number of words circled.

4. Determine the approximate grade level from the chart below.

SMOG Conversion Table

Total Polysyllabic Words	Approximate Grade Level (+ or - 1.5 grades)
0 - 2	4th
3 - 6	5th
7 - 12	6th
13 - 20	7th

Figure 1. READABILITY TESTING. McLaughlin, G.H. (1969). SMOG - A new readability formula. JOURNAL OF READING, (May), 639-646.

PICTORIAL EXAMPLE FOR PERSONS WITH LOW LITERACY SKILLS

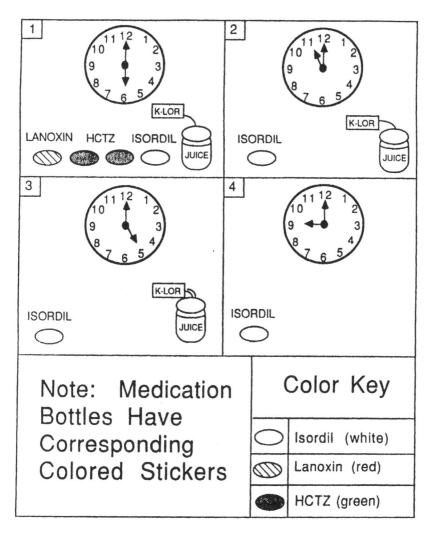

Reprinted with permission of Aspen Publishers, Inc.
From Dunn, M., Buckwalter, K. & Pilti, H. (1985).
Teaching the illiterate client does not have to be a problem.
Family and community Health, 8, p.79.

APPENDIX C

SAMPLE CARE PLAN USING COGNITIVE, AFFECTIVE, AND PSYCHOMOTOR DOMAINS

Teaching Plan for Sublingual Nitroglycerin Tablets

Assessment	Plan/Learning Objectives	Interventions	Evaluation
	COGNITIVE DOMAIN		
Ask the client/family what they know about angina.	Client/family will list the beneficial effects expected from tablets.	Give client/family fact sheet on proper storage, effect, and use of tablets.	Ask client/family to explain effect, use, and strange of the medication.
Ask the client/family what they know about using nitroglycerin tablets.	Client/family state how the nitroglycerin tablets are to be administered, when and how many.	Show client, family the tablet and explain how they are given and discuss the scheduling.	Ask client/family to tell you when the client is to use the tablet and show you how many.
Ask the client/family what they know about risk factors associated with angina.	Client/family will list risk factors associated with angina and which ones should be reported to physician or nurse.	Give client/family list of information on risk factors and how to get in contact with a health professional.	Ask client/family to explain and list the risk associated with angina and what to do if symptoms occur.

AFFECTIVE DOMAIN

Ask client/family about concerns they have regarding taking nitroglycerin. (What have they heard from other people?)	Client will ask about concerns or problems e.g. feelings about side effects from nitroglycerin.	Let client discuss feelings without being judgmental. Correct misconceptions without discounting client's concerns.	Client shares feelings about nitroglycerine side affects and reports both times that have been taken and when has omitted them.
Ask client/family to express fears or concerns about angina.	Client win discuss feelings about effect that angina has on personal life and ability to function.	Give client information on how to reduce stress and ways to alter life style taking into account client's fears.	Client reports use of ways to reduce stress and is consistent in taking action to reduce episodes of angina.

PSYCHOMOTOR DOMAIN

Observe/record use of nitroglycerin tablets and refill history.	Client will keep a record of symptoms and use of nitroglycerine.	Provide method of record keeping or help client develop one.	Clients demonstrates ability to keep accurate records. Records number of pills taken, symptoms and if relieved.
Observe/record progress in changing habits that increase angina.	Client will exercise, maintain normal weight, and not smoke.	Provide with information about groups that help with supporting health.	Client uses tablets correctly and maintains healthy lifestyle.

Adapted from Kloeppeik, J., & Henry, D. (1987). Teaching patients, families, and communities about their medications. In c. Smith (Ed.) Patient Education: In partnership with other health professionals. Orlando, FA: Grune & Stratton, Inc., pp., 293–295

MINI-MENTAL STATE

Maximum Score	Client Score	
		ORIENTATION
5	___	1. What is the (year) (season) (date) (day) (month)?
5	___	2. Where are we (state) (county) (town) (street) (number)?
		REGISTRATION
3	___	3. Name three objects: (e.g. cat, ball, rose). Then ask the client to repeat all three after you have said them all. Give 1 point for each correct answer. Then repeat them until he/she has learned all three. Count trials and record. # of Trials _____
		ATTENTION AND CALCULATION
5	___	4. Serial 7's. Ask to subtract 7 from 100 (93, 86, 79, 72, 65). If does not get any of serial 7's right then ask to spell WORLD backwards (DLROW 0-5) and score it instead. If the person can not understand the word world due to poor hearing substitute another five letter word.

RECALL

6. Ask for the 3 objects repeated in number 3. Give one point for each correct answer.

3 _____

LANGUAGE

7. Show the client a pencil and a watch and ask "What is this?" (2 points).

2 _____

8. Ask the client to repeat the following: "no ifs, ands, or buts" (1 point)

1 _____

9. Following a 3 stage command. "Take a paper in your right hand, fold it in half, and put it on the floor." (3 points). Another 3 stage command may be substituted if person unable to do task due to physical impairment.

3 _____

10. Have the client read and obey the following:
   CLOSE YOUR EYES (1 point)
   WRITE A SENTENCE (1 point)
   COPY THE DESIGN (1 point) Draw a circle, square, and triangle. Ask client to copy them. Tremor or shakiness ignored but all three must be closed figures.

3 _____

TOTAL
SCORE   _____
(30)

Figure 2. Mini-Mental State. Folstein, Folstein, & McHugh (1975); adapted.

APPENDIX D

RESOURCE SUGGESTIONS FOR TEACHING OLDER ADULTS

Recommended for Home Care Staff

BOOKS

Doak, C., Doak, L, & Root, J. (1985). Teaching patients with low literacy skills. Philadelphia: J.P. Lippincott Co. (170 pages - Price $10.95).

This book is a must for any home health agency library. It is a 170 page paperback with many illustrations on how to approach the person with low literacy skills. It provides pictures and illustrations of how to adapt reading materials, audio tapes, and vocabulary to be comprehensible to persons of varying verbal abilities. Tests are provided and how to use them in a sensitive way for determining the reading level and understanding of vocabulary by patients in any setting. A final chapter is on teaching persons with learning disabilities.

Loustau, A. (1986). Health promotion and patient teaching. In M. Patrick, S. Woods, R. Craven, J. Rokosky, & P. Bruno. Medical surgical nursing: Pathophysiological concepts (pp. 42-48). New York: J.P. Lippincott.

Although this is written in a medical-surgical text, it is equally applicable for home care. It is a short concise well written chapter with illustrations of concise teaching plans to aid a home care persons is gaining a quick grasp of teaching principles and how to apply them with clients. The textbook is large but a reprint of the chapter could be obtained from a nursing school near by, it is a quick and helpful reference for any agency staff member involved in teaching adults.

Smith, C.E. (Ed.) (1987). Patient education: Nurses in partnership with other professionals. New York: Grune & Stratton, Inc. (363 pages - Price $29.50)

This is an excellent text for patient teaching and is recommended for any teaching library. It has practical short chapters on teaching and provides continuity from chapter to chapter with illustrations of nursing care plans that are tailored to teaching. The plans are concise and outcomes are easily grasped. It is as practical for home teaching as it is for hospital teaching. The well written chapters are based on research but are written with the clinician in mind with short chapters and easily understood brief care plans.

PERIODICAL ARTICLES

Hallburg, J.C. (1976). The teaching of aged adults. Journal of Gerontological Nursing, 2 (3), 13-19.

This article, though almost ten years old, is still consistent with current literature in reviewing aspects of teaching that need to be adapted for the aged.

Kane, R.L., Kane, R.A, & Arnold, S.B. (1985). Prevention and the elderly: Risk factors. Health Services Research, 19, (6, Part II), 945-1005.

This is an excellent well researched article written by physicians and has excellent tables for a review of important health risks and illnesses and their frequency in older populations. It is an valuable resources for selection of topics for health promotion and education. The information provided is enough to motivate both the teacher and older adults to be informed about the topics.

Rendon, D., Davis, K, Gioliella, E. & Tranzillo, M. (1986). The right to know the right to be taught. Journal of Gerontological Nursing, 12, 33-38.

This article is specific to teaching elderly. It is directed to a nursing home population, but is equally applicable for home care. It presents model and concise organization of factors to take into account when teaching the elderly.

Tideiksaar, R. (1984). Guidelines for teaching the adult learner. Physicians Assistant, (Dec), 46-53.

This article is well written and concise with neat tables that summarize adaptations for the adult learner.

Recommended for Developing Programs for Older Adults

Brandts, W. & Hooyman, N. (1982). A Manual of Psychosocial Issues and Community Resources for the Elderly. Seattle, WA: Institute on Aging and The Long-Term Care Gerontology Center. (53 pages - Price $5.00)

This is a manual of ways to help family caregivers by using available resources. It is written primarily to alert physicians to home care issues with resources available in the Seattle area. It could serve primarily as a guide for setting up such a manual for local physicians and health agencies.

Family Seminars for Care Giving: Helping Families Help

A Facilitators Guide and A Participants Handbook. Available through Institute on Aging: University of Washington JM-20, Seattle, WA 98195. The Facilitators Guide is $29.95. The participant handbook is going out of print and a close out offer is being made of $7.00.

This is an exact content and teaching method guide for setting up seminars for family care givers of older chronically ill members. It can be taken as developed and used by any home care agency or mental health agency to establish a care giving support group. Individual sessions could easily be used for community wide education on the subjects provided. Six sessions are described in detail and each could be used over several sessions. The subjects include (1) Changing roles and relationships; (2) Communication and decision making within the family; (3) Health issues associated with aging; (4) Community resources; (5) Getting through the day - includes how to get along with difficult impaired older adults; (6) Common concerns of the caregiver - includes legal issues as well as how to take care of yourself.

Gray, M, Kethley, A., Kiehn. J., Rose, C. (1981). <u>Neighbor Helping Neighbor</u>
<u>Volunteer Program.</u> (A Manual for Training and Program Replication).
Seattle, WA: Institute on Aging (81 pages - Price $11.50)

This is a detailed manual on how to set up a Neighbor to Neighbor
volunteer program. The program's purpose is to promote helping
behaviors among the elderly through education on how to be good
helpers and use community and medical resources appropriately.
The manual trains volunteers to go out and teach the elderly these
skills. A section is provided on training the teachers and then the
content and specific instructions are provided for the volunteers who
teach other elderly persons.

Hooyman, N., & Lustbader, W. (1986). <u>Taking Care: Supporting Older</u>
<u>People and Their Families.</u> New York: Free Press. (324 pages - Price
$24.95.

Complete with charts and information sheets such as a medical bill
accounting sheet, a task delegation sheet for family meetings, a
phone recording sheet for locating community services and
transportation, plus a cost comparison of long-term alternatives, this
resources can be used by both professionals and families.

Montgomery, R., & Prothero, J. (Eds.). (1984) <u>Developing Respite Services</u>
<u>for the Elderly.</u> Available through University of Washington Press,
P.O. Box C-50096, Seattle, WA 98145 (206) 543-4050. (82 pages -
Price clothbound = $20.00: Paper bound = $8.95.

O'Connor, K., & Prothero, J. (Eds.). <u>The Alzheimer's Caregiver:</u>
<u>Strategies for Support.</u> Available through University of
Washington, P.O. Box C-50096, Seattle, WA 98145

<u>Family and Client Resources</u>

Mace, N., & Robins, P. (1981). <u>The 36-hour Day: A Family Guide to</u>
<u>Caring for Persons with Alzheimer's Disease, Related Dementing</u>
<u>Illnesses and Memory Loss in Later Life.</u> Baltimore:
John Hopkins University._(Price $3.95]

Pacific Northwest Extension (1984). <u>Aging Parents: Helping When Health</u>
<u>Fails.</u> Oregon State University Extension Service: PNW 246.
(Price $1.25)

Pacific Northwest Extension (1985). <u>Families and Aging: A Guide to Legal</u>
<u>Concerns.</u> Oregon State University Extension Service: Extension
Circular 1221. (Price $1.25)

Pacific Northwest Extension (1985). <u>Helping Memory- Impaired Elders: A</u>
<u>Guide for Caregivers.</u> Oregon State University Extension Service:
Extension Circular 1211. (Price $1.25)

Pacific Northwest Extension: These three guides are 12 to 20 pages in
length and are excellent resources to give to families to read.

Silverstone, B., & Hyman, H.K. (1982). <u>You and Your Aging Parent.</u>
New York: Pantheon. (Price $8.95)

This book is excellent for adult children of the chronically ill
elderly. It is easy reading and provides important information
with case examples that keep the reading easy. Family relationships
as well as ways to understand the formal care system are provided.

Task Force on Aging (1987). <u>How to hire a helper: A guide for elders and
their families</u>. Seattle, WA: Church Council of Greater Seattle
Can be ordered through the church council at 4759 - 15th Ave N.E.,
Settle, WA 98105; (206) 525-1213

This 12 page booklet sells for $3.00 with a reduced rate for
quantities. It has been in demand since its initial publication
two years ago. There are a few telephone numbers in it specific
to the Seattle area, but it can be used as a model for hiring
helpers in any location.

Places to Obtain Additional Client Education Materials

American Cancer Society
219 East 42nd Street
New York, New York 10021

American Diabetes Association
18 East 48th Street
New York, New York 10017

American Foundation for the Blind
15 West 16th Street
New York, New York 10011

American Heart Association
44 East 23rd Street
New York, New York 10010

American Lung Association
1740 Broadway
New York, New York 10019

National Association for the Deaf
814 Thayer Avenue
Silver Springs, MD 10910

National Association for the Visually Handicapped
305 East 24th Street
New York, New York 10010

National association of Hearing and Speech Agencies
814 Thayer Avenue
Silver Springs, MD 20910

APPENDIX E

Contributors' Biographic Information

Barbara Horn, R.N., Ph.D.
Principal Investigator
Professor, Department of Community Health Care Systems SM-24
School of Nursing
University of Washington
Seattle, Washington 98195

Anne Loustau, R.N., Ph.D.
Associate Professor, Department of Physiological Nursing
Assistant Dean, Academic Programs
School of Nursing
University of Washington
Seattle, Washington 98195

Kathleen O'Conner M.A.
Editorial Consultant
190 Queen Anne Avenue North, 3rd Floor
Seattle, Washington 98195

Betty Pesznecker, R.N., M.N.
Co-Principal Investigator
Associate Professor, Department of Community Health Care Systems SM-24
School of Nursing
University of Washington
Seattle, WA 98195

Martha Worcester, R.N. Ph.C.
Gerontological Nurse Practitioner
School of Nursing SM-24
University of Washington
Seattle, Washington 98195

Chapter IV

Family Coping:
Caring for the Elderly in Home Care

Martha Iles Worcester, PhC

Principal Author

Patricia Archbold
Barbara Stewart
Rhonda Montgomery

Consultants

Kathleen O'Connor, MA

Editing

SUMMARY. This paper focuses on the nature and significance of family caregiving problems when providing assistance to chronically ill or frail older adults. It includes theoretical frameworks that provide explanations of related research about family coping problems, a guide for assessment of family caregiving problems, and a summary of current findings relative to home care agency planning and health care policy. The Family Caregiver Assessment Guide for use in home care agencies is included in the appendix to the paper.

This paper is a portion of the material developed by the project staff of the Elderly Home Care Project, Principal Investigator, Barbara J. Horn. Funded by Fred Meyer Charitable Trust. Sponsoring agency: University of Washington, Department of Community Health Care Systems, Seattle, WA 98195.

121

INTRODUCTION AND OVERVIEW

Families who care for elderly ill or frail family members has become a major area of research interest as well as a concern for home health agencies. The reasons for the increase in interest are due primarily to the convergence of three major changes. The first is the fact that there are an increased proportion of elderly persons in the population needing to be cared for by families. The second is that the health care system is now able to manage chronic illness so that people live longer during some of their frailest years thus extending the time that families and the formal care system are involved in providing care. The third and most recent change is the increased cost of health care which has resulted in the earlier discharge of older persons from acute care settings along with more stringent criteria for reimbursement of both home care and nursing home utilization.

With these changes families are experiencing the need to care for ill or frail elders more often, for longer periods of time and in both acute and long term chronic illness.

This chapter addresses the extent and nature of the caregiving experience for families and presents an assessment guide to be used for aiding home care agencies in assisting families to cope with the care of ill older family members in the home.

The first part of the chapter is an overview of the magnitude of the caregiving experience within the United States and expected trends in the future. The second section contains a review of the literature on the types of problems families must confront within the course of caring for an older ill member. The discussion provides four perspectives for viewing caregiving. They include: (a) family responsibilities assumed; (b) the burden experiences; (c) the role changes that take place; and (d) the nature of support provided by kin, friends, and the formal system of care.

The third section is a presentation of an assessment and planning guide and the method by which it was tested and revised in collaboration with home health agencies. The final section summarizes the current state-of-the art and its relevance for home care agency planning and social policy.

Background and Purpose

This paper was written in a response to a need identified by staff in home care agencies that participated in the Elderly Homecare Project (Horn, 1986). The project was funded for a period of three years (1986 to 1989) by the Fred Meyer Charitable Trust and administered through the University of Washington, School of Nursing. It was designed to identify and provide approaches to clinical problems that home care agencies experienced with the earlier discharge of the elderly from hospitals.

In order to identify the problems the home care agencies faced, a survey was conducted of 178 Medicare certified home health agencies in the Northwest region of the United States. Of the 118 agencies responding, 87.5 percent reported that management of family coping problems, secondary to the acute condition of patients on discharge from the hospital, was a major problem. The survey indicated that staff identified family problems with coping, as stress, fear, apprehension, anxiety, burnout, fatigue, weakness, and feelings of being overwhelmed. These feelings were often attributed to two problems: (a) the families' lack of understanding or knowledge of needed care, and (b) the lack of community or family resources that could help family members cope or have time away from caregiving. The amount of nonreimbursable time nurses spent helping families manage the health problems of the recently hospitalized older person also was reported as problematic for agency budgets. This time included the difficulty staff had in assessing and dealing with the emotional impact of the elder's illness on family members, and finding interventions that would enable the family to retain their independence while coping with the caregiving process.

Some coping difficulty for families was attributed to the caregiver's functional inability to perform the physical care required. These factors have been more adequately addressed under specific types of physical care needs that will be discussed within other papers and clinical approaches to be developed by this project. This paper will focus on the issues with which families must cope as they assume the care of an impaired older member.

The Importance of Family Caregivers

It is common knowledge that the proportion of people over 65 years of age in the United States is increasing and is expected to reach 30 percent of the total population by the year 2030. This figure is based on the present population, and is adjusted for current life expectancies (NCHS, 1984). These statistics have major implications for the role of the family in caregiving when older members become ill, frail, or incapacitated. Although 5 percent of the frailest elderly are in institutional settings, at least twice as many are equally disabled and are being cared for in the community. Of the elderly in the community who need care, 80 percent are cared for solely by their families, 12 percent seek care from informal caregivers, and only 8 percent use formal systems of care at any point in time (Gurland et al., 1983).

The number of persons residing outside of institutional settings who require help with basic activities of daily living, increases with age: between ages 65 to 74 — 2 percent need help; ages 75 to 84 — 14 percent need help; and ages 85 and above — 40 percent need help (Feller, 1983). The fastest growing segment of the population is the over 85 age group. The average life expectancy at 85 is 6.7 years (NCHS, 1984, section 6, Table 7). Thus, the frailest group is not only becoming more numerous and living longer, but is also increasing at a faster rate than the care providing group (U.S. Bureau of Census, 1982).

The decreasing proportions of those who provide care is not often realized. When looking at 20 year increments from 1920 forward, the ratio of persons (ages 45-65) who are in the group providing care to the elder (ages 75 and over) care-receiving group has decreased from 11:1 in 1920; 9:1 in 1940; 8:1 in 1960; to 5:1 in 1980. Projections based on current life expectancy show a continuing decrease from 3:1 in 2000 to 2:1 in 2040 (U.S. Bureau of Census, 1982). These demographic changes come at a time when social policy is calling for decreased expenditures for the aged, as well as shortened hospitalizations for their acute care. Families and home care agencies are expected to care for elders in increasing numbers at a time when numbers of family members available are decreasing. In addition, care is expected of families in more acute phases of illness while reimbursement sources have cut the amount alloted for family home services.

Brody (1985) outlined a historical perspective to the cost and toll that spouse and parent caring imposes on families as social programs begin to withdraw support and give even more responsibility to families for care of elders at home. Brody views the proportions of elders needing care and the extension of life for the disabled elderly as an entirely new phenomenon. The growth of research on caregiving is a direct response to the added proportion of families who assume a caregiving role to parents or spouses for extended periods of time.

UNDERSTANDING FAMILY CAREGIVING: CONCEPTS AND RELATED RESEARCH

As a basis for understanding the research literature and nursing assessment pertaining to caregiving, it is helpful to review some of the current theories and concepts that have provided a framework for research efforts and explanation of results. Family theory, burden, role theory, social networks and social support are a few of the most relevant models. A thorough understanding of these theories and concepts would require greater discussion than presented here. A brief introduction and definition of terms precedes the following research summaries relevant to each model.

Family Theory

There are many definitions of family that help describe family purpose and function. One such definition has been chosen to provide a context in which to view the family. Terkelsen's (1980) traditional definition is presented here.

> A family is a small social system of individuals related to each other by reason of reciprocal affections and loyalties and comprising a permanent household (or cluster of households) that persist over years and decades. Members enter through birth, adoption or marriage and leave only by death. (p.23)

The family's purpose is to provide a context in which the survival and developmental needs of all its members are supported. Family

tasks are most commonly expected to include: (a) physical maintenance of its members; (b) socialization and maintenance of family
members for roles within the family and other social groups; and (c)
maintenance of social control within the family and between family
members and outsiders (Terkelsen, 1980). Although this traditional
definition and purpose does not take into account all ethnic and life
style differences, it does clarify the expectations that most societies
commonly have of the family.

Family Care of Elders Research

Research about family care of its aged members has been primarily descriptive rather than directed at intervention. In response to
the long standing popular myth that families are decreasing their
care for aged members and abandoning them to nursing home care,
many studies have been conducted to determine if such a trend exists. Extensive literature reviews (Doty, 1986; Streib & Beck, 1980;
Troll,1971) revealed that families do not abandon their elder members and continue to provide for their care even in the face of increased mobility of families and more extended periods of necessary care. In a study of nursing home admissions, it was found that
50 to 60 percent of clients admitted had no living children and of
those who did, considerable care had been provided prior to admission (Brody, 1982; Streib & Beck, 1980). Even when institutionalized those residents with family members still were visited frequently (Brody, 1981; Soldo & Myllyluoma, 1983).

In the past it was considered rare to care for an elder member, but
the current increase in survival rates of elders now means that it is
common for adult children not only to assume the care of parents,
but to also care for more than one parent at a time or a series of
parents over the years. The developmental stage of family life in
which parent-caring occurs varies, but most often begins in late
middle age (ages 55-65). Usually these caregivers are women who
also lose spouses during this time. In addition, due to the trend in
deinstitutionalization of all ages and types of handicapped and mentally ill individuals, families may be caring for parents at the same
time as caring for adult children that have not been able to leave
home due to handicaps (Brody, 1985). When numerous difficulties
must be dealt with by the family at one time or over a short period

of time, McCubbin et al. (1980) appropriately term this as "a pile up of life events."

The belief in the commoness of three generational households in the United States is another widely held myth. In fact, research has shown that, not only in the United States, but also cross culturally, multigenerational households have been highly unusual. In the past, when families did assume the caregiving role for an older member, it was usually for a short time since people died at younger ages or from more acute illnesses. The norm has been, and continues to be, that each generation wants to maintain a separate residence, and usually does, until infirmity of the aged necessitates a common household (Nydegger, 1983).

Empirical evidence indicates (as summarized by Litwak, 1985) that there are three stages of family proximity as elders age. First, in their 60s, or when elders are healthy, they tend to live at some distance from kin and in age homogeneous communities. Second, in their 70s, they tend to move close to kin or into the same household if care demands are great. Finally, in their mid or late 80s, or with increasing disability, they move into institutions if care demands become too great for family members to manage at home. However, there are major class and ethnic differences to this predominant trend.

In summary, research on the family as caregivers of elders has shown that families not only do care for elder members, but are doing so despite the need for increasing lengths of time for which care must be given, the increasing amounts of care needed, and the increasing numbers needing their care. The following burden literature discussion is a first step toward describing the impact on the family of caring for an ill adult in the home setting.

Burden Research and the Nature of Caregiving

The concept of burden, as experienced by family caregivers, originally developed in Great Britain in the 1960s in response to the deinstitutionalization of the mentally ill. Physicians were concerned that patients treated in the community setting would be too much of a burden on families. The first series of studies conducted attempted to determine if the burden experienced by families whose members were discharged earlier and treated as out-patients was greater than that of families whose members were treated with the traditional longer periods of institutional care (a situation not unlike the earlier discharge of the medically ill today). Later studies arose from concern for family caregivers of impaired elders and therefore are directly related to the Elderly Homecare Project concerns.

The concept of burden was first defined as "how much effect" the patient's illness had on family income, employment, leisure activities, domestic routine, children in the home, health of household members, and relationships with neighbors as judged and rated by the interviewer (Grad & Sainsbury, 1963,1968). In that study 60 percent of the families experienced an impact on the mental health of household members, 35 percent experienced disruption in their leisure and social activities and 29 percent experienced alterations in their daily routines. The level of burden was rated by the interviewer on a three point scale. "Some" burden (a rating of 2) was experienced by two thirds of the 410 family sample.

Hoeing and Hamilton (1967) classified burden into objective and subjective components. The effects on household life and the patient's abnormal traits were defined as objective burden, whereas a global rating of burden defined the subjective component. The significant finding from the study was that 81 percent were judged by the interviewer to have significant objective burden but only 60 percent of the families reported subjective burden.

Herz, Endicott, and Spitzer (1976) added symptoms of family members to the objective indicators of burden, and included such items as "have trouble sleeping." One hundred and seventy-five families of patients were followed for 24 months after the patient was admitted to a psychiatric program. The patients were divided into three treatment groups with varying degrees of family responsibility for patient care. Although no differences in amount of burden related to the treatment was reported by families, 62 percent of all the families reported subjective burden that included worry about the future.

Platt and Hirsch (1981) divided objective and subjective burden more distinctly. Objective burden was considered to be concrete events, happenings, and activities, whereas subjective burden was defined as feelings, attitudes, and emotions. A group of 224 patient families were divided into out-patient and in-patient treatment groups. Again, no significant differences were found in amount of burden based on type of treatment. The most common types of objective burden were adverse affects on the family member's physical and emotional health, as well as stress related to the patient's behavior, the patient's poor social performance, and arguments within the family concerning the patient's behavior.

In the 1970s and 1980s, literature related to burden began to address caregivers of the dependent elderly in both the United States and Great Britain. In Great Britain, Sanford (1975) found that 12 percent of geriatric hospital admissions were related to the family caregivers' feeling that they were unable to manage the patient's care. On interviewing these family members he asked them what factors had to be alleviated in order to restore a tolerable situation at home. Sanford found that the least tolerated behaviors of the patients were those that resulted in sleep disturbance for the primary caregiver (62 percent). Sleep disturbance was caused by night time wandering, the patient's inability to get on and off the commode unaided, and irrational shouting. Another frequent and poorly tolerated behavior (43 percent) was fecal incontinence while urinary incontinence was well tolerated. In 46 of the cases (92 percent) families could identify the specific behaviors that, if alleviated, would permit the elder to return home. Only four family caregivers (8 percent) said they would not take the elder home under any circumstance. Though the word burden was not used in this study, its findings suggest an approach to determining what must be changed for a family to be able to decrease the burden enough to continue homecare.

In 1980, Zarit, Reever, and Bach-Peterson defined burden as feelings of discomfort or concern with respect to the psychological well-being, financial situation, and social life of the caregiver. They therefore, limited their definition of burden to the subjective component of burden. In a sample of 29 elderly persons with senile dementia and their family caregivers (18 spouses and 11 daughters), caregivers reported feelings of anger, embarrassment, guilt, pain, suffering, fear, depression, strain and discomfort. The most frequently reported items eliciting these emotions were loss of personal time and fears about future deterioration of the care-receiver's behavior. The important findings stemming from this study were that the patient's level of functional disability did not relate to the feelings of burden of the caregiver, nor did the duration of the illness. However, caregivers who received more visits from family members perceived less burden.

The influence of the duration of the illness (e.g., whether burden increases, decreases or remains constant over time), has also been studied, but the findings are inconsistent. In studies by Grad and Sainsbury (1968); Hoeing and Hamilton (1967); and Johnson and Catalano (1983), burden was found to increase or persist over time. These studies involved collection of data extending over four year periods. In two to five year studies conducted by Robinson and Thurnher (1979), it was found that there were phases of increased burden, but over time the difficulty of caring for elders increased and intensified. Both the Herz, Endicott and Spitzer (1967) and the Gilhooly (1984) study, however, reported a decrease in feelings of burden over time but neither study specified the length of time over which the data was collected.

Thompson and Doll (1982) coined the affective dimension of burden as "emotional cost" and used burden to encompass feelings of overload, feeling trapped, resentment, and exclusion (wanting to escape or get away from the ill family member). Objective burden was defined as "disruptions in every day life" as a result of caring for the ill family member. Of the 125 families in the study, 72 percent expressed feelings of being overloaded, 42 percent expressed feelings of being trapped, and 40 percent expressed feelings of resentment. The most frequent type of objective burden reported (50 percent) was the constant supervision required by the patient.

In a study conducted to determine if chore services reduced family caregiver burden, Montgomery, Gonyea, and Hooyman (1985), defined objective burden as "the extent of disruption or changes in various aspects of the caregiver's life and household" (see Appendix A). Subjective burden was defined as the caregiver's "attitudes toward or emotional reactions to the caregiving experience." This study found that there was no relationship between caregiving tasks and subjective burden, but that there was an increase in objective burden related to caregiving tasks that required the caregiver to be available most of the time (e.g., tasks of bathing, dressing, and walking the care-recipient).

In 1984, Poulshock, and Deimling presented another framework for burden which viewed the impairments of elders as a causal factor in determining feelings of burden (i.e., tiring, difficult, or upsetting). It analyzed the impact of these feelings on the household. Zung's Depression Scale (Zung, 1974) was used for the first time in this study to determine if burden was associated with depression. The results indicated that impairments of the care receiver involving disruptive behavior or interfering with social relationships, were most consistently associated with feelings of burden. Depression was only slightly related to how restricted the caregiver felt about caregiving. It was not clear however, whether the depression caused the restriction in social relationships or vice versa.

It was obvious that the various meanings assigned to burden were not comparable among the various studies. Major differences arose: (a) burden being what was observed versus what was experienced by the person in the situation; (b) burden being described as an event, versus the result of an event; and (c) burden being described as care that was needed versus reactions or attitudes toward having to provide the care.

However, despite the discrepancies in models and the differences in the instruments used to measure burden, some consistent results emerged. Montgomery, Stull, and Borgatta (1985) provided a useful summary in a literature review. A major theme, validated by many sources, was that what was defined as objective burden (symptoms of patients, functional ability of patients, lack of environmental resources) was not directly related to subjective burden. As Montgomery and Associates noted, what one person viewed as requiring little assistance and, therefore, not at all burdensome, might be the basis for another person requiring a great deal of assistance and be perceived as very burdensome.

What the burden literature indicates, is a need to define burden clearly and to separate objective burden (that which can easily be observed) from subjective burden (that which is a part of the caregiver's reactions to the events). Currently, subjective burden is being defined more consistently as the reactions (usually feelings) to the events, symptoms, or environment of caregiving, while the events are viewed as objective burden. Subjective burden encompasses caregivers' feelings of resentment, guilt, fear, and anger and

descriptions of caregiving activities as upsetting, difficult, and trying. Objective burden encompasses the number and types of activities that must be performed (Zarit, Reever, and Bach-Peterson,
1980; Poulshock and Deimling, 1984).

Table 1 summarizes and classifies burden factors into demographic factors, care-receiver impairments, caregiver reactions, and
impact on family life. The Table notes those factors which contributed most to feelings of burden across several of the studies.

Although the burden literature has contributed a great deal to

TABLE 1. Factors Contributing to Family Caregiver Burden

1. DEMOGRAPHICS

    age
____sex
    income
    education
    physical environment

2. CARE-RECEIVER IMPAIRMENTS _____

    Physical and functional
    problems
    mobility
    urinary incontinence
    * ability to get to
      commode unaided

    Mental and behavioral problems
    * disruptive behavior
    poor social performance
    * night time wandering

3. CAREGIVER STRAIN

    Physical Health
    * trouble sleeping____

    Mental and Emotional
    Health
    intolerance of
      incontinence
    * intolerance of being
      awakened at night
    feelings of
      * resentment
      * being trapped
      * being overloaded
      being angry
      * embarrassment
    * guilt
      fear, strain
      suffering
      discomfort
      depression

4. IMPACT ON FAMILY LIFE

    trouble with neighbors
    * social isolation
    arguments about patient
    financial cost
    * loss of personal time

    * loss of leisure time
    * disruption of everyday
      routine
    constant supervision
      of ill elder
      required

"*" items are those which were found to be in common across
several studies.

describing some of the difficulties of caregiving and the caregiving impact on family life, the inconsistency of the scales measuring burden across studies, the different terms used to define burden, and the variability in classification of factors that influence burden, have rendered the research findings vague. The studies involving the mentally ill did not detect a difference in burden for families whose members were hospitalized for short periods of time versus those whose members were hospitalized for a longer period of time. However, these studies also did not identify who the caregivers were (i.e., daughters, husbands, or wives), nor did they note whether or not the mentally ill member was newly diagnosed or had been having problems for a long time prior to inclusion in the studies.

The other major problem with burden studies has been the implied, but not clearly stated, relationship of burden to outcomes. The implication exists that if caregiver burden is less, then the impaired person should need shorter periods of institutional care. The other consideration that is implied, but not tested, is that home care of the ill person will not unduly affect the health of the caregiving family or the care-recipient any more than would be the case under traditional longer periods of in-patient care. A model of relationships of the burden factors to such outcomes is presented in Figure 1. This model implies that demographic factors such as age, sex, marital relationships and income and the type and amount of care-receiver impairments, produce effects on family life and result in caregiver reactions such as burden. Therefore, amount of burden experienced will then influence the length of time the caregiver will be able to provide care and the physical and mental health of the caregiver and care-recipient.

Role Strain and Caregiving

Role Theory and Role Strain

The caregiving role and expectations of persons in that role are other factors that have been examined. Role theory presents a readily understandable method of viewing behaviors of caregivers and their families. In role theory the "role" is defined as a set of prescriptions defining what the behavior of a person should be in

Factors Influencing Burden	Burden		Potential Outcomes
Demographic Factors	Objective:	Disruptions in family life	Length of family caregiving
Care-receiver Impairments	Subjective:	Caregiver perceptions	Caregiver Health Care-receiver Health

FIGURE 1. The Effects of Factors on Burden and Potential Outcomes for the Caregiver and Care-receiver

relation to other persons in a given context (Burr, Leigh, Day, & Constantine, 1979). The status or position of a role refers to how each person is related to another (e.g., mother to daughter, boss to employee). Role strain is one of the more relevant concepts in role theory and is often used to explain the stress that occurs as a result of caring for older family members.

Role strain is defined by Goode (1960) as "the felt difficulty in fulfilling role obligations." According to Burr (1979), some of the most influential factors that determine the amount of role strain are consensus about role expectations between those involved, the amount of reward in engaging in the role, and the ability to compartmentalize different roles. Thus, a caregiving spouse or daughter experience role strain when it is difficult to comply with the role expectations set by others or themselves, when there is little reward received from engaging in the role, and when there is difficulty keeping caregiving from interfering with other roles.

Research and Role Strain

Types of role issues that will be used as a basis for understanding the next set of research studies will include gender roles, family roles, role reversal, role ambiguity, role confusion, role demands, role conflict, role overload, and role expectations. Gender differences in caregiving roles have been researched by Horowitz, 1985; Robinson and Thurnher, 1979; and Seelbach, 1977. These studies found that the woman's role of health care supervision was considered the norm. Responsibilities in caregiving that were commonly assumed differed for the man and the woman. A woman viewed her responsibilities as those of personal care and "making the parent happy," while a man saw his role as advisory or providing financial or care management support. The woman often felt a great deal of guilt if the parent was unhappy, while the man did not assume responsibility for the feelings of the parent. Both the husband of a caregiving daughter and the daughter's male physician, therefore, frequently counseled the adult daughter to become "less involved with the parent" (Robinson & Thurnher, 1979). In addition, if the caregiver was male (whether son or spouse), more help was solicited from outside the family or in the case of the male son, from his spouse than was the case when the caregiver was female.

The nature of the family role, in respect to the care-recipient, also varied in the type of responsibility assumed in the caregiving role. If the caregiver was a spouse and female, more personal care was provided with less support from within or outside the family. However, if the caregiver was a daughter, care was either provided by the daughter or the daughter organized the services to be provided for the parent. When role reversal occurred this often added to the strain experienced. Thus if the spouse-caregiver was male, the woman's traditional role of caregiver was reversed. Role ambiguity and role confusion were often the result.

The parent-caring role has also been described as role reversal between parent and child. In fact it is truly a new role and has thus contributed to role confusion. Although the nurturing and caring-for elements of the child-caring role might be similar, the actual ways of relating in a parent-caring role are very different because of the prior mother-daughter relationship. In addition, as Goldfarb (1965) reflected, caring for an infant entails the expectation of increasing independence, while caring for the older adult indicates an increasing dependency and need for assistance by the care taker. Also, when caring roles have been reversed from the past, the caregiver and care-receiver have more difficulty in meeting mutual expectations (Archbold, 1980), thereby increasing role strain. The fact that less role strain is often reported by spouse-caregivers than by daughters who care for parents, when the same amount of care is given, is explained by the spouse-as-caregiver being more a part of role expectations by the culture, while there has been less precedent and role modeling for the daughter in the parent-caregiving role (Johnson & Catalano, 1983).

The role demands of caregiving, as enumerated by Archbold (1980), included preventing medical crises, controlling symptoms, carrying out treatment regimens, preventing social isolation, adjusting to the disease course, attempting to normalize life, and finding the necessary resources and money to provide care — all in the interest of the parent. Encroachment on the family's or caregiver's time and future plans (Clark & Rakowski, 1983), along with role conflict and role overload that is induced by competing roles (e.g., spouse, mother, employee) or too many tasks to accomplish within one role, was found to compound the difficulty in the caregiving role and decrease the morale of caregivers. Role demands that are not complimented by some rewards also contributed to a decrease in the caregiver's morale — as when care recipients were demanding or unappreciative or could not communicate due to aphasia (Brody, 1981; Fengler & Goodrich, 1979).

The type of caregiving demands, as reported by Archbold (1982 & 1983), often differed as to whether one took on a care providing role or a care management role. Care providers (those who did all the care themselves) usually lived with the care-recipient, had daily care demands and experienced restriction of personal time, and constant daily irritation. The care manager (those who managed the provision of care by others) usually lived in a separate residence, and also had full time jobs. The care managers experienced more time limitations outside of work time, less career mobility, and a financial drain. Caregivers in both provider and manager roles experienced guilt for not doing enough.

Role expectations often added to the strain in several ways: (a) when role expectations of the caregiver and care-recipient did not match (i.e., the care-receiver demanded more than the caregiver thought was needed or the reverse, Archbold & Stewart 1986); (b) when the caregiver thought he/or she should do more; (c) when parent-caring was demanded of a retired couple who both were expecting increased personal time and leisure (Cantor, 1983); and (d) when family members disagreed as to the amount of care other family members should give to the impaired elder.

The model that follows (Figure 2) summarizes the following factors that have been shown to influence role strain. In the Figure, the roles expected due to gender and family relationships lead to role ambiguity and role confusion when roles are reversed or persons lack prior positive experiences in the care giving role. Role demands differ depending on whether the caregiver provides the care or manages the care, and role conflict and role overload are created when the caregiver must also be involved in work or has other family commitments. When demands of the caregiving role are great and the care-recipient is not able to communicate, there may be few rewards received by the caregiver. Role expectations create more

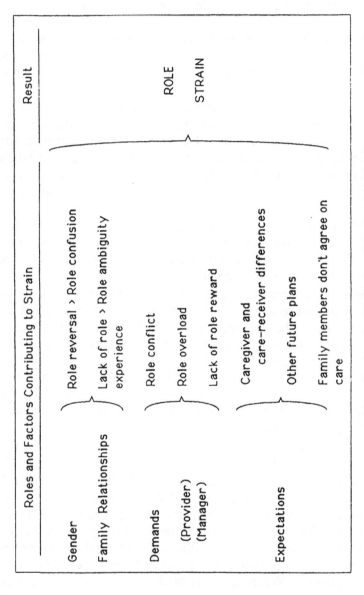

FIGURE 2. Factors Contributing to Caregiver Role Strain

strain when the caregiver and care-receiver do not agree on the amount of care needed and when the caregiver had different future plans than those permitted when providing care. All of these factors together influence the perceived amount of role strain.

Social Support and Social Networks

Concept Definitions

Concepts of social support and social network have been used to help determine if those elderly with smaller social networks or fewer aspects of social support are more vulnerable to institutionalization (Brody, 1982) or have higher rates of formal services use (Chappell, 1985). In Cassel's (1976) and Henry's (1982) study, better social support and more developed social networks were associated with increased resistance to disease (e.g., by altering physiological mechanisms such as endocrine balance through neocortical input from the environment). Thus, social support and adequate social networks were seen as buffers against life stress. Because stress, strain, and burden have been used interchangeably in much of the caregiving literature, and have been viewed as having negative effects on the caregiver, reduction of such stress through better social support has been a major emphasis in programs developed for caregivers.

Concepts of social support and social network have a broader application focus than the care-recipient and caregiving family. Social support refers to the way in which the person is receiving help from family, other people, agencies, and environmental resources. The most common definition of social support is:

> Interpersonal transactions that include one or more of the following: "affect" (expressions of liking, admiration, respect, love), "affirmation" (expressions of agreement of rightness of some act or statement of another person), and "aid" (transactions in which direct aid or assistance is given — including things, money, information, advice, time and entitlement). [From Kahn & Antonucci (1980) as cited in Broadhead et al., p. 529 (1983)]

Social network, on the other hand, refers to the number, frequency and linkages between contacts with other individuals or groups (McKinley, 1981). Litwak, in *Helping the Elderly* (1985), proposed a structure for viewing social networks to determine sources of the various aspects of social support just defined. Social networks were defined as:

a. Primary groups – that include the marital household, kin, close friends, and neighbors;
b. Informal groups – that include self initiated groups (e.g., self-help or personally hired, non-agency help), volunteers, and friendship groups; and
c. Formal groups – that include agencies in the community, and institutional settings.

Litwak considered not only the aspects of social support and the classification of social networks, but also examined the characteristics of those social networks in relationship to such characteristics as proximity, quantity, and linkages between types of support for the persons who used them. These three dimensions: (a) aspects of social support; (b) type of social network; and (c) characteristics of the social network, provide a useful framework for discussion of the research literature that follows. An illustration of the way the three dimensions fit together is presented in Figure 3. The type of group and example of aspects of social support comprise the first two dimensions. An example of the third dimension (Network Characteristics) would be how close the person or agency is that provides the support, how many people are included in that type of support and how well the types of support are linked together for ease of utilization.

Research Related to Concepts of Social
Support and Social Network

Research projects relating to caregivers' use of support systems, and programs developing better support for in home care of the elderly, have been based, in large part, on the untested assumption that the rate and use of expensive institutional care can be reduced for elders with chronic long term impairments or acute conditions

FIGURE 3. Aspects of Social Support and Network Characteristics According to Type of Social Network

TYPE OF SOCIAL NETWORK	ASPECTS OF SOCIAL SUPPORT				NETWORK CHARACTERISTICS		
	Aid (examples)	Affect (examples)	Affirmation (examples)		Proximity	Number	Linkages
Primary	personal care time	love concern	assurance that the way care is given is appreciated				
Informal	transportation yard work		agreement that care of elder is important				
Formal	skilled nursing care		assurance that care is done correctly				

141

by increasing primary network support, informal network support, and formal home care support (Branch & Jette, 1983). The findings of these studies and programs comprise the following discussion.

Primary, informal, and formal networks have been examined to determine the characteristics of caregivers who use different types of networks, as well as the types of social support these networks provide. Studies have consistently validated that caregivers preferred to use primary and informal networks whenever possible (Branch & Jette, 1983; Stoller & Earl, 1983). Spouses and daughters who lived with the care-recipient tended to provide all aspects of social support more often than other persons who were part of the care-receivers' primary network (Stoller & Earl, 1983). Use of informal supports increased when the functional ability of the care-recipient decreased (Kohen, 1983), but it was also found that caregivers in residence (most often spouses) might also decrease both family and informal contacts as care demands increased so that social isolation often became pronounced (Fengler & Goodrich, 1979; Silliman, Fletcher, Earp, & Wagner, 1986). Both men and women, however, turned first to their children (usually daughters) when they were having difficulty providing all of the needed care (Kohen, 1983).

Adult children (particularly widowed women) who were caregivers had more informal network resources than did spouse caregivers and used them more readily for care support. However, when decision-making on behalf of the ill elder was required, caregivers consistently relied on themselves and a few close family members to make decisions and did not include informal or formal care networks as participants (Townsend & Poulshock, 1986). In research done by Scott and Roberto (1985), proximity was found to be the most important factor in determining the use of primary and informal networks. If family or kin lived within an hour of the care-recipient, most of the care was usually provided by those family members.

The existence of a primary network, however, did not always mean that the network was socially supportive to caregivers. Several studies demonstrated that primary networks added to the stress of caregiving if family members were in conflict over what care was needed (Archbold, 1983; Johnson & Catalano, 1983). Good relationships between the caregiver, siblings, and other family members were found to be associated with better morale of the caregiver.

In a representative sample of 1625 noninstitutionalized elderly, Branch and Jette (1985) found that the kind of care needed was another factor considered in the type of support network used. When choosing between primary or informal networks and formal networks for caregiving tasks, the family and informal groups most often provided all of the basic care needs (e.g., assistance with bathing, dressing, eating, and grooming), while formal networks were used for more instrumental needs (e.g., assistance with housekeeping, transportation, and grocery shopping). The findings of Litwak (1985) supported the theory that proximity, the nature of the task, and the kind of services provided by formal agencies were factors that determined the type of network used.

Age was also found to be a factor in use of formal networks for care. Comparison of groups of care-recipients from 75 to 84 years of age with the group over 85, showed an increase in the use of formal support services. Use of formal care services for basic care needs increased from 20 to 40 percent and for instrumental needs from 72 to 99 percent. Formal services offered to support caregivers of ill elders have been studied to determine if they reduce the stress and burden of caregiving or if they reduce the likelihood of the care-recipient needing institutional care. Formal support services that provide home health aides, chore services, respite care, mutual support groups for caregivers, and case management programs are the types of services that have been examined. The research results concerning such programs follow.

In a study by Brody, Poulshock, and Masciocchi (1978), it was found that the living arrangement of the care-recipient was much more influential in whether institutionalization was necessary than the presence of a home health aide. If the care-recipient lived with the caregiver, caregiving was extended for a longer period of time than if the caregiver lived in a separate residence. Thus, it was considered to be more important to evaluate the influence of the family care unit than to expect that adding a home health aide (HHA) to the caregiving would prevent institutionalization. Home health aides were helpful, but it was recognized that the HHA was only a small part of the care that was being provided.

Another study, by Hooyman, Gonyea, and Montgomery (1985), examined the effects of withdrawing chore services to determine if caregivers who had chore services, perceived less stress and burden than those who had chore services discontinued. Interviews of 42 relatives of clients who had services discontinued and 38 clients who had continuing chore services were asked whether burden or stress were increased or decreased over the prior year. No differences could be found between the two groups. A thorough examination of the results found that families did not do any less for the care-recipient whether they did or did not receive chore services.

The findings indicated that chore services were additions to what was being provided, and the family was already doing the maximum it could when chore services were offered. In addition, chore services had not been providing care that was usually associated with what was most burdensome for families (e.g., chore services provided help with yard work, shopping, and meal preparation while caregiving tasks that were most burdensome for family caregivers were bathing, personal care, and feeding). Most chore services were also provided in small amounts (from 1 to 4 days a month) and, in conjunction with other help. Thus, chore service could not be shown to reduce the amount of burden or stress in a measurable way, even though such services were reported by caregivers to be very helpful.

One multi-service support program offered for older women caring for disabled husbands at home, was developed through the wives' self initiated support group (Crossman, London, & Barry, 1981). It incorporated case coordination, adult day care, home care, and extended respite care. Caregivers reported that weekend out-of-home respite care for husbands was particularly helpful in reducing the stress of intense caregiving and that being out of the home also raised the mood of their disabled husbands. These effects could be viewed as enhancing the positive feelings (affect) and appreciation (affirmation) of care-recipients toward their caregiving spouses.

In the Crossman et al. program, wives experienced less guilt on leaving their husbands when the home care or respite provided was done by a professional versus other formal care providers. Adult day care services were found to be helpful, but at times, the stress and effort required in getting the husband ready to go counter balanced the relief from caregiving during his absence. If the husband was attending adult day care, having the same personnel provide in-home respite care increased the acceptance of the in-home respite for both the disabled spouse and the wife giving care. Services provided by the program were not studied to determine if they prevented use of institutional care. It was suggested by the advocacy group formed by the wives, however, that studies should to be done to determine how many women who were in nursing homes were there due to the physical and emotional effects of prolonged caregiving to husbands.

Mutual support groups provided through community home health agencies, were viewed as an important means of providing social support for caregivers by Pesznecker and Zahlis (1986). These groups provided forums for problem-solving within the group and informal networking outside of the group's time. Affective support was established through shared experiences and feelings, and therefore diminished the negative emotions of anger, resentment, and guilt. Aid, or instrumental support, was provided through sharing ideas about how to approach problems and exchanging information about community resources, legal issues, and financial resources. The affirmation aspect of social support was provided by the positive reinforcement members gave each other about their caregiving efforts and their own importance as individuals.

For the groups to be successful in providing the three aspects of social support, certain guidelines were considered important for conducting and facilitating the group. A set of rules was developed to cover issues of:

a. Confidentiality;
b. The right of each member to have time in every meeting to share personal experience; and
c. The attitude that advice was to be helpful and not critical, and members could accept only what was useful to them.

By reading such rules at the beginning of each meeting, the group learned how to be supportive and new members were easily integrated. Members who dominated the meeting, or who were too demanding of the group, could be referred to more individual types of supportive services. The studies found that it was important to focus more on the caregivers' own frustrations and feelings and ways to alleviate them, than on finding solutions to caring problems for the care-recipient.

Coffee breaks, in these groups, were found to be good times for building informal networks of support. The professional-facilitators could gradually withdraw their involvement and let the family caregivers assume more and more of the tasks of organizing and leading the group. Consequently, a formal system of support could be transferred to an informal system or network. Although it was felt that the facilitator should be available as a resource person should the group need it in the future, the mutual support group could be seen as a means of strengthening informal support networks. Whether or not such a service could indirectly impact the cost of long term care remains untested.

In an analysis of twelve support programs for family caregivers, it was found that they provided education, problem solving skills, mutual peer support, and reduction of negative feelings associated with caregiving (Clark and Rakowski, 1983). However, across all programs, objectives were rarely stated and outcomes measured were limited. Measurements of program effectiveness included anecdotal comments by participants, leader observations of the group, questionnaires that tested knowledge of information presented in the groups, and self esteem scales.

Case management is a special type of social and network support that involves assigning one person to determine how all possible services will be provided to a client. Case management is usually regarded as important for better coordinated care (e.g., better linkage of primary, informal and formal networks) of socially supportive programs.

A large comparative study of five different types of case management programs, focused on determining what type of case management might be least costly and most effective in reducing the need for institutionalization of the elderly (Capitman, 1986; Capitman, Haskins, & Bernstein, 1986). Across the five programs in five different sites (New York City; San Diego, California; South Carolina;

and two sites in San Francisco) there was a wide range of cost due to factors that were not directly related to the case management approach. Types of services available, types of clients, types of reimbursement of services available to clients, and use of specialized professionals versus persons with less educational background for case managers were all factors that affected the cost. However, case management programs that restricted agency use were found to be the least costly.

Although one program did show a decrease in nursing home use, this program was more restrictive in its admission policies to nursing homes. It was suggested that the finding—that the four other sites did not reduce use of nursing homes—was due to nursing homes already being restrictive in admissions and below the level of what is really needed by the community. One finding was that better functional ability of the care recipient did not reduce the rate of nursing home use, but the existence of and availability of informal support did. It was concluded that with the low rate of use of formal systems of care that now exists, it is probably not feasible to reduce costs, but that programs need to be provided that foster a better quality of life than now exists under the current system of care.

As demonstrated in the prior discussion, formal support networks must consider many factors related to providing resources for older families. Several home care agencies in the Elderly Homecare Project reported that for those who needed a lot of care in the home, it was often necessary to have many different workers (e.g., nurses, physical therapists, health aides, and chore workers) during the week, which was difficult for home care agencies to coordinate, as well as difficult for those in the patient's household to tolerate. However, most home care agencies found that there was just not enough formal support available to relieve caregivers.

An area that is part of social support, but is not usually considered within its domain, is community and nation wide policy regarding formal system services. This is an area that received the most comment from the survey conducted by the Elderly Homecare Project and is currently a topic of debate in the research literature. Recent research demonstrates that shortened hospital stays increase the need for home care agency services (Beebe, K., Callahan, & Mariano, 1986; Guterman, & Dobson, 1986; Taylor, 1985). The

Elderly Homecare Project survey confirmed those findings, and found that, due to earlier hospital discharges, acute health care needs in the home took more time resulting in an inability to meet the needs of the chronically ill elderly. For some communities, resources were adequate to meet the increased demands, but for most there were not enough staff or financial reimbursement mechanisms available for necessary care.

The research of support programs reviewed above are outlined in Table 2 and Table 3. Table 2 presents the types of networks and the aspects of social support that apply to each. Table 3 reviews the characteristics of the networks that influence caregiving. Both supportive (+) and non-supportive (−) features of the networks and aspects of social support are included.

By exploring the types of social networks and social supports that are part of the caregiver's environment, a more complete picture is provided than would be possible by just considering burden and role strain. Actual sources of support can be identified and thereby services can be planned that are complementary to the care already being provided. Other family members and informal networks that are within the proximity and already linked with the caregiver can become important supports when home care provided by formal agencies is lacking or has limited resources.

Summary of Family Caregiver Difficulties

Although concepts related to family theory, burden, role theory, and social support networks were all useful to understanding and organizing certain aspects of caregiver difficulties, no one framework contains all the caregiver difficulties that need to be addressed. Therefore the most frequently occurring problems in providing care that have been identified in the prior literature review, are now classified under four categories to present a comprehensive picture. These categories include: (a) the tasks required by the caregiver; (b) the caregiver's physical and mental well being, (c) the effect of caregiving on the caregiver's life style: and (d) the effect of caregiving on the caregiver's social network (see Table 4). A summary of the specific problems under each of these categories is presented in the Table 4. The problems summarized in the table served as the background for the development and testing of a caregiver assessment and planning guide. The purpose, development, description, and field testing of the guide follows.

THE CAREGIVER ASSESSMENT AND PLANNING GUIDE

Development and Purpose of the Guide

A proposed assessment guide, derived from major concepts in the literature, was presented to experts in academic and home care settings for critique of the purpose, the format and content, and decisions as to the methods of testing the guide. The subsequent statement of purpose for The Caregiver Assessment and Planning Guide (CAPG), the format of the guide and the procedures for testing the guide are the results of these combined efforts of faculty and clinicians.

The central purpose of the CAPG is to provide home health professionals with the necessary information for determining specific areas for which family caregivers need assistance from the home health agency, and in what areas caregivers are able to manage the care alone or with assistance of family or friends. The guide was developed primarily for use in the home setting by nurses and social workers of home care agencies. The CAPG is to be used for:

a. Identifying caregiver abilities and problems in independently managing the care of an impaired elder;
b. Prioritizing and planning interventions; and
c. Evaluating the effectiveness of those interventions.

In the following discussion the guide is described, the methods by which it was tested, the results of the testing, and a discussion of the results. The Caregiver Assessment and Planning Guide is presented in the form in which it was tested in Appendix A.

Description of the Caregiver Assessment and Planning Guide

The guide (see Appendix A) was developed to be used with the person who provides the most care for an older ill or frail family

TABLE 2. Types of Social Support for Family Caregivers of Elderly

TYPES OF NETWORKS	ASPECTS OF SOCIAL SUPPORT		
	AID	Affect	Affirmation
Primary Networks Spouses Daughter sons Close friends	+ Basic ADL Instrumental ADL Decision-making Acquiring formal services - Health problems of caregiver reduces aid	+ Caring, love, worry affection - Resentment anger, conflict	+ Encouragement, appreciation - Disagreement over way care is given
Informal Networks Self-initiate Volunteers Personally hired	+ More often instrumental ADL Basic ADL Advice Problem-solving Require more supervision and recruiting time		+ Raise self esteem, encouragement - May increase stress if focus on negative

Formal Networks	+	+	+
Home health	Basic & skilled care	Expression and resolution of stressful feelings	Sense of self worth
Chore service	Instrumental ADL	Enhances positive feelings	Belief in abilities
Mutual support groups	Information (financial, legal resources, advice)		Restores belief in importance
Respite care	– Periodic relief from all caregiving		
Case management	Can improve access to all forms of service and help		
	–	–	–
	Adult day care may increase stress due to difficulty in getting care-recipient ready	Poorly led mutual support group may increase feelings of resentment and	If members of mutual support group are judgmental, caregiver may feel inadequate
	Case managers may limit access to needed services		

ADL = Activities of Daily Living:
"+" = supportive features of the network
"–" = non-supportive features of the network

151

TABLE 3. Characteristics of Social Networks and Their Relationship to Caregiving and Social Support

CHARACTERISTICS OF SOCIAL NETWORKS OF CAREGIVERS

Proximity

1. The closer the proximity of the primary or informal network the more likely that network will be used for support.
2. Those who live with the caregiver most often provide the greatest amount of support.

Quantity

1. Smaller caregiver networks are more vulnerable to relinquishing the caregiving responsibility and to institutionalization of the care-receiver.
2. The smaller the caregiver network, the more likely that help will be needed from formal networks.
3. The more care that is required, the more likely that the caregiver will become isolated from primary and informal network contacts.
4. Caregivers who are widowed or single women with few family members are more likely to have more and stronger informal networks.
5. Too many types of professionals in the home from formal agencies are likely to decrease the supportiveness of the help provided.
6. Too many different types of formal agencies offering services decrease the supportiveness of the care provided.

Linkages

1. The more highly educated the caregiver the more linkages she/he will have between primary, informal and formal networks.
2. Mutual support groups increase linkages with informal networks.

member. During the subsequent discussion the Caregiver Assessment and Planning Guide can be referred to in Appendix A.

Section I: Identifying Information

This section contains basic information about the caregiver (e.g., sex, age, who to contact in an emergency). Only minimal information is included about the care recipient because the CAPG is intended to be kept with the care recipient's chart in order to prevent unnecessary duplication of information.

TABLE 4. A Summary of Caregiver Difficulties

A. Caregiving Tasks Required and Ability to Manage Them
    1. Lifting care-receiver
    2. Managing urinary or bowel incontinence
    3. Night time problems of care-receiver that keep caregiver awake
    4. Managing care-receiver disruptive behaviors or emotional problems
    5. Dealing with hearing or sight deficits
    6. Complicated health regimen's or technology (e.g. many types of medications to give or IV equipment in the home)

B. Caregiver's Physical and Mental Well-Being
    1. Inadequate sleep
    2. Health problems not being treated
    3. Persistent fatigue and weakness
    4. Increase in taking medications for nerves and/or sleep
    5. Weight loss of more than 5 pounds in the last two months
    6. Poorer physical health
    7. Feelings of being overwhelmed by the situation
    8. Feelings concerning the inability to provide care.

C. Effect on Caregiver's Lifestyle
    1. Isolation from usual activities
    2. Unable to find time away from caregiving
    3. Difficulty finding time to meet other responsibilities to family, friends, and/or jobs
    4. Disruption in family life
    5. Restrictiveness of caregiving

D. Social Network and Social Support
    1. Decrease in contacts with family and friends
    2. Difficulty in finding help from family and friends, others
    3. Decrease support from family and friends over time
    4. Differing expectations of caregiver by the care-receiver and by formal or informal helpers
    5. Family or friends often too far away to help
    6. Difficulty coordinating help from health care resources
    7. Reluctance to ask family or formal sources for help

---

*These are an integration of the literature previously reviewed including Archbold & Stewart 1986; Brody 1985; Cantor 1983; Clark & Rakowski 1983; Robinson 1983; Robinson & Thurnher 1979.

Section II: Essential Questions for the First Visit

These are questions that need to be asked of the caregiver on the first home visit or preferably, prior to discharge of the care receiver from the hospital. They include questions about the caregiver's ability to do the care needed and knowledge of how to obtain help in emergencies, the presence of other family members that might be able to help with providing care, and financial concerns related to obtaining services.

Section III: Problem Identification

This section is divided into part A and part B. Part A asks about what assistance the caregiver must provide the care receiver and part B asks the caregiver about what effect the caregiving is having on his or her own physical, psychological, or social well being. In both part A and B, the caregiver is asked to answer yes or no to each question and then rate the level of difficulty of the item on a four point scale with 4 being very hard, and 1 being easy. The rating scales are for aiding the clinician in prioritizing problems at the time of the initial assessment. Later, the ratings are used to determine if the intervention decreased the level of difficulty in relationship to the problem for which it was intended. Thus, if "lifting" was a problem and instruction was given on moving and lifting the care receiver, the rating for lifting should show a decreased level of difficulty. Likewise, if "feeling isolated and alone" was rated high, then attendance at support groups and provision of respite to provide time to be with friends should decrease the level of difficulty in dealing with that problem. In addition to evaluating the effectiveness of interventions, the guide can be used intermittently to reassess the changing concerns of the caregiver.

Section IV: Major Stresses, Strengths, and Support

The assessment of major stresses and supports contained in Section IV focuses on what the caregiver views as the primary concern and strengths and sources of support. Interventions can then be planned that use resources already available or to provide resources consistent with the caregiver's preferences (e.g., if the caregiver is feeling frustrated because there is no time for activities other than caregiving and views the church as his or her main support, respite for attending church activities might be the most helpful).

Section V: Plan of Care

The final section of the CAPG (V. Plan of Care) provides space for listing problems and actions to be taken and directly corresponds to the problems identified in prior sections. The items in the prior sections are listed as numbers with their rating followed by the intervention that is planned (e.g., Section III A #8: Rated 4 — Talk with physician about reducing the number of medications).

Field Test of the Caregiver Assessment and Planning Guide

The overall objectives in testing the guide were (1) to determine its effectiveness in identifying and prioritizing caregiver needs and (2) to plan interventions to meet those needs. More specific objectives were: (a) to determine whether the questions were easily understood by family caregivers; (b) whether the clinicians found the format easy to follow: and (c) to determine the time it took to complete the assessment.

Sample

Two urban clinical agencies participated in the testing the guide. One was a small hospital based agency and the other was a large independent home health agency. Five clinicians in each home care agency volunteered to test the guide. Informed consent was obtained from each of the volunteers after they were given both written and verbal explanations of the study.

Eight nurses and two social workers participated in the study. Their experience in the agency ranged from 1 to 17 years with a mode of 2 years. The nurses educational background included one with an Associate Degree, two diploma program graduates, and. five with Bachelors Degrees. The social workers both held Master's Degrees.

Each clinician was instructed to use the guide with five family caregivers of the agency's elderly clients (65 years old and over). Each of the clinicians interviewed five family caregivers, resulting in the guide being used with a total of 50 family caregivers. The caregivers' ages (displayed in Table 5) indicated that a majority of

TABLE 5. Caregiver Ages* N = 50

AGES	NUMBER	PERCENT
20 – 39	4	8
40 – 59	7	14
60 – 69	13	26
70 – 79	17	34
80 – 85	7	14
Missing	2	4

caregivers were over 60 years of age with 14 percent over 80 years of age. Of the caregivers 28% (14) were male and 72% (36) were female. The caregiver's relationship to the care recipient was spouses (60%), and adult children (26%) with the remaining caregivers either siblings (6%) or other relatives or friends (8%).

Procedures

Participating clinicians were given a half hour orientation to the CAPG. This orientation consisted of a brief explanation of how to use the guide and a role playing practice session. In the role playing session, one clinician conducted the assessment and one played the role of a caregiver. An opportunity for questions and answers was provided after the role playing session. A sample of a completed assessment form was also provided to participants.

The participating clinicians were also asked to complete an evaluation form to be used each time a CAPG was completed (see Appendix B). The evaluation form contained instructions for the participant to rate the CAPG on a scale of 1 (poor) to 5 (excellent) as to the how well the caregiver understood the questions, clarity of each section of the CAPG, and the helpfulness of the guide in identifying ways to support the caregiver. The length of time it took to fill out the guide and any comments the participant would like to make concerning the form were also requested.

After completion of all the CAPGs and their respective evaluation forms, one final overall evaluation form was requested (see

Appendix C). The participants were instructed to return the completed CAPG along with the evaluation form by mail in a preaddressed and stamped envelope the day the assessment was done. The quantitative information (e.g., ages of respondents, and rating scales) were computer coded and entered for analysis. Content analysis was conducted on the open ended questions of the CAPG, and on the comments requested in evaluation forms.

Findings: Response Rate

All of the Caregiver Assessment and Planning Guides were completed and returned resulting in a one hundred percent response rate. Of the evaluation forms attached to each CAPG, 45 of the 50 forms specific to each guide were returned for a 90% response rate, and all of the final overall evaluation forms were returned. In the following data analysis, the results from the CAPG forms are presented first, followed by responses of participants to the evaluation forms.

Findings: CAPG

Section I of the guide was "Identifying Information." Age, sex, and relationship of the caregiver to the care-recipient were part of this section. The ages of caregivers are reported in Table 5. Of the caregivers, 30 were spouses (17 wives and 13 husbands), 12 were daughters or daughters-in-law, and 3 were sisters. The remainder were more distant relatives (3) and in one instance a neighbor. Section II of the guide is not discussed here because in the evaluation of the guide, clinicians reported that this information was repetitive of information already acquired through routine assessments.

The caregivers' responses to sections III and IV reported here have been selected to provide examples of the type of information that was obtained. As stated previously in Section III of the CAPG, caregivers were asked if the problem existed and then asked to rate the problem as to the difficulty they had in dealing with it. Levels of difficulty were rated 1 to 4, with 4 being the most difficult. The reported frequency and mean difficulty level of caregiver problems are presented in Table 6.

Management of the care-recipient's behavior problems was the

TABLE 6. Caregiver Problems and Level of Difficulty

III.A - PROBLEMS IN PROVIDING CARE	# REPORTED (N = 50)	%	DIFFICULTY (1 - 4)*
1. Management of behavior problems	29	58	3.04
2. Managing medical equipment	29	58	2.07
3. Checking on at night	28	56	2.08
4. Lifting	27	54	2.82
5. Bowel problems	27	54	2.40
6. Managing medications	25	50	2.44
III. B - EFFECT ON CAREGIVER			
1. Feelings of isolation	35	70	2.79
2. Fatigue and weakness	35	70	2.57
3. Feeling overwhelmed	31	62	3.27
4. Trouble getting sleep	30	60	2.58
5. No time away from care	28	56	2.63

* This is the mean level of difficulty. The caregiver was asked how difficult was this problem for him or her and asked to rank it as: 1 = easy; 2 = not too hard; 3 = pretty hard; or 4 = very hard. The total number of caregivers assessed was 50.

most frequently occurring problem reported by caregivers (29 times — 58%) and was also rated as most difficult with a mean of 3.04. "Feelings of isolation" was the most frequently reported effect of caregiving on the caregiver's life (35 times — 70%) with a mean level of difficulty of 2.97, second in difficulty to " feelings of being overwhelmed" (mean of 3.27).

At the end of Section III A and B caregivers were asked if there were other problems that had not been included. Personal care problems (e.g., bathing, dressing, and feeding the care-recipient) were the types of problems most frequently added as other problems.

The content of the responses by caregivers to the open ended questions in section IV of the CAPG were analyzed and organized into categories according to central themes. The four major themes in answer to the effect caregiving had on their own lives (see Section IV #3 and #5 of the CAPG) were (a) interruption of their own personal time and other role responsibilities, (b) difficulties in providing and managing the physical care required, (c) difficulties in dealing with the negative attitudes and behaviors of the care recipient, and (d) difficulty in dealing with their own feelings related to caregiving. Examples of exact statements made by caregivers in each of these categories and the frequency with which items occurred within the category are presented in Table 7. When caregivers were asked about the way they managed their problems and concerns (see Section IV, #4 and 6 of the CAPG) the themes that characterized their responses were: (a) get away for awhile or do other things; (b) be with or talk to other people; (c) rely on my faith; and (d) maintain a positive attitude (see Table 7 for examples). When asked who they relied on for support, family members was the most frequent response (60 times). Friends and home health agency personnel were reported 14 times each.

The Plan of Care (Section V) as filled out by clinicians, was the final section of the CAPG. The responses were analyzed and categorized by the same method as the other open ended responses. Teaching and referral were the two most predominant interventions listed in the Plan of Care. Forty-one different teaching interventions were suggested. Nineteen concerned teaching the caregiver to manage the care-recipient's symptoms, six consisted of teaching about the care-recipient's disease, and four concerned teaching about medication management. The remainder were specific to care-recipient problems (e.g., catheter care, relaxation techniques for the caregiver, colostomy care).

The most frequent referrals made were to the social worker (38 times). Eleven referrals were made without specifying a reason. Making arrangements for respite was designated as a reason for ten of the referrals. Chore service, support groups, meals on wheels, financial concerns, and changing the living arrangements were each named three times as the reason for referral. Eleven other referrals were mentioned as needing to be arranged without specifying the

TABLE 7. Caregiver Responses Regarding Stresses (N = 50)

QUESTIONS AND RESPONSES   FREQUENCY

Question: <u>What do you find most stressful or difficult</u>
           <u>about caregiving?</u>

A. Interruption of personal time & role responsibilities (22)
   "no time for activities I enjoy" - "life is disrupted"
   "don't like being away from home"
   "the time involved and scheduling it takes"

B. Providing and managing the physical care required   (21)
   "keeping all the medications straight"
   "figuring out what to cook that she will eat"
   "lifting him"

C. Dealing with the negative attitudes and behaviors of
   the care-recipient   (15)
   "she has such a stubborn attitude"
   "he is demanding and cranky" - "his depression"
   "she is not able to cooperate due to memory loss"

D. Dealing with feelings related to caregiving   (11)
   "I feel so helpless" - "I worry about what will
    happen next" - "facing that he will never get well"
   "having to ask friends for help"

Question: <u>What helps in relieving the stress?</u>

A. Getting away for awhile or doing other things   (30)
   "spending less time there" - "taking a break"
   "working on projects" - "going shopping"
   "sitting down" - "resting"

B. Being with or talking to other people   (34)
   "just having other people come to visit"
   "talking with other family members"
   "visit with friends"

C. Relying on my faith   (21)
   "religion and prayers" - "I am a believer that God
   can do anything" - "I go to church and read the
   Bible daily" - "my faith"

D. Maintaining a positive attitude   (18)
   "laughter, and concentrating on the positive
   aspects of life and simple pleasures"
   "hearing about other elderly people who have
   recovered" - "trying to be optimistic"

social worker as the person to arrange them (e.g., hospice, dietitian, enterostomal therapist). In the Plans of Care it was also noted that a variety of services suggested to the caregiver were refused (19 times).

Although the original intent of the guide was to link the information acquired from the caregiver to a specific intervention in the plan of care, this was not done in any of the Plans of Care. Rather, several interventions were listed together at the end and their connection to the specific items had to be inferred.

Findings: Evaluation Forms

The results of the evaluations of the CAPG by the clinicians are reported next. The mean ratings for ease of filling out the form and client's understanding of the form were 3.8, and 3.3 respectively with ratings on a 5 point scale (1 = poor and 5 = excellent — see Appendix C). The mean length of time for filling out the CAPG ranged from 35 to 90 minutes with a mean of 35 minutes. There was no significant difference in the ratings or length of time for completing the CAPG form between the two agencies.

Suggestions for changing the form included; (a) making it more concise, (b) adding more items related to personal care, and (c) combining questions on major stresses. To make the form more concise, participants suggested that Section II be eliminated as this information was already being collected. In Section III it was suggested that the "occasionally" option be omitted (see Section III, column 2).

Clinicians suggested questions needed to be added about personal care (help with toileting, dressing, eating and bathing). These items were consistent with those which had been added by the caregivers in the blanks provided for "other problems" that had not been included on the list in Section III A of the CAPG. The fourth section on major stresses (see CAPG, Section IV) had included items that asked the caregiver "what produced the most stress" and "what produced the most difficulty." Comments on evaluation forms from clinicians were that clients said these questions were repetitive. Rewording and simplification of the questions were suggested.

Discussion

As stated earlier, the objectives of testing the guide were (1) to determine its effectiveness in identifying and prioritizing caregiver difficulties and (2) planning interventions to ameliorate those difficulties. Section III of the guide was the most definitive in identifying caregiver difficulties. The information was specific and the caregivers were able to designate the degree of difficulty. The responses were consistent with the research literature on caregiver stresses and strains (Brody 1985; Cantor 1983; Clark & Rakowski 1983; Robinson 1983; Robinson & Thurnher 1979) thus lending content validity to the items selected for problem identification. Section IV's open ended responses supported the Section III's most frequent responses and priorities. For example the feeling of lack of time for any activities other than caregiving (the most frequent response as a major stressor in Section IV) can be logically associated with the feelings of isolation reported most frequently in Section III. The two most frequent ways of dealing with stress — "getting away for awhile" and "being with or talking to other people" — supports the need for interventions such as respite and support groups.

The Plan of Care, Section V, was the weakest section of the guide. This section was not linked to specific items nor was there any mention of which items should be given first priority. There may have been several reasons for the weakness of this section. The orientation was brief and even though an example of a completed form was provided, more time was given for how to do the assessment and no practice time was provided for writing the Plan of Care. Another likely explanation is that the Plan of Care required additional time outside the interview, and participants had work priorities that took precedence over completing the guides.

Of the interventions reported, the most frequent was teaching with a focus on teaching the caregiver to deal with the physical problems of the care recipient. The referrals for respite or chore services did not match the frequency of the reported stress of lack of personal time or the expressed need by caregivers to get away for awhile. The unspecified referrals to social workers may have been for this purpose. An additional factor that provides some explanation for the lack of match between the types of problems reported and types of interventions, was the number of times all suggestions for outside assistance were refused (19), particularly interventions related to respite or support groups. Such refusals are consistent with findings in the caregiving literature. For example when respite or support groups are suggested, it takes a great deal of encouragement by the clinician to convince caregivers that time away is beneficial for their own health and therefore indirectly for the health of the care recipient (Montgomery, 1985; Clark & Rakowski, 1983).

As a result of the way in which the CAPG guide was used and the critique of the guide by clinicians, the guide has been revised to be more concise, less repetitive of information already collected, and to increase the likelihood of linkage of interventions in the plan of care to responses of caregivers (see Appendix D—Proposed Revision of the Guide). The major revisions include:

a. Elimination of Section II of the CAPG
b. Elimination of "occasionally" as a response in Section III of the CAPG
c. Revision of question in Section IV under major stressors
d. Numbering all items consecutively for ease of reference to prior items in the plan of care.

Clinical Applications of the CAPG

To make the best use of the revised form the most important aspect is practice in use of the form that includes writing the plan of care as well as in collection of the information in Sections I through IV. When used appropriately, the form can aid in setting priorities for reducing caregiver stresses. The rating scales of Sections II and III can be used at the first contact with the caregiver and in periodic assessment of the caregiver to serve as a measure of goal attainment (e.g., decrease in the difficulty rating scale after an intervention for that difficulty) and to determine which interventions are most effective in reducing caregiver difficulties. Finally, if clinicians across many settings can continue to collaborate with researchers in futher development of the guide, results of caregiver responses can be analyzed and used to provide direction for program planning specific to the needs of caregivers.

CONCLUSION

Given the context of current home care practice, evaluation of and interventions for caregivers are considered to be time consuming and non-reimburseable. Only skilled care and education reimbursement categories can be used to denote time given to caregiving assessment. Unfortunately there is no reimbursement available to home care agencies for time spent with the express purpose of interaction (other than education) with the caregiver. Some monies are being provided for limited respite care, but many restrictions apply.

Arguments can be offered that without such assessments and timely intervention, the caregiver and care-recipient will ultimately need more expensive institutional care. However, these arguments must be proven to national policy makers in order for adequate resources to be developed. With increasing demands on families to provide more acute care, as well as long term chronic illness care for older family members, it is even more critical for formal health care agencies and educational centers to develop effective assessment and interventions methods.

As the proportion of the population needing care increases, more resources will be needed for both in home and institutional care. Researchers concur (e.g., Archbold, 1982; Litwak, 1985; Hooyman, Gonyea, & Montgomery, 1985), that family and informal networks have absorbed the maximum caregiving responsibilities that should be expected in a society that can afford to offer more alternatives if there was better planning and priority setting.

Better assessment and intervention plans can be developed with continued communication between health practitioners and educators so that research findings can be made relevant and practical for the clinical setting. Developing reliable and uniform assessment tools and field tested interventions can, in turn, provide the information needed for national health policies that are responsive to the needs of caregivers and their families.

REFERENCES

Archbold, P. (1980). Impact of parent-caring on middle-aged offspring. *Journal of Gerontological Nursing, 6* (2), 78-85.

Archbold, P. (1982). An analysis of parent-caring by women. *Home Health Care Services Quarterly, 3* (2), 5-25.

Archbold, P. (1983). Impact of parent-caring on women. *Family Relations, 32,* 39-43.

Archbold, P., & Stewart, B. (1986). Preliminary report of caregiver relief study. Consultation conference with Elderly Homecare Project University of Washington, School of Nursing.

Beebe, K., Callahan, W., & Mariano, A. (1986). Medicare short-stay hospital length of stay, fiscal years 1981-1985. *Health Care Financing Trends, 3* (1), 119-123.

Bradburn, N. (1969). *The structure of psychological well-being.* Chicago: Adeline Publishing Co.

Branch, L., & Jette, A. (1983). Elders' use of informal long-term care assistance. *Gerontologist, 23,* 41-56.

Brandt, P., & Weinert, C. (1981). The PRQ—a support measure. *Nursing Research, 30* (5), 277-280.

Broadhead, E., Kaplan, B., Janes, S., Wagner, E., Schoenbach, V., Grimson, R., Heyden, S., Gosta, T., & Gehlbach, W. (1983) The epidemiologic evidence for a relationship between social support and health. *American Journal of Epidemiology, 117,* 521-537.

Brody, E.M. (1981). Women in the middle and family help to older people. *Gerontologist, 21,* 471-480.

Brody, E.M. (1985). Parent care as a normative family stress. *Gerontologist, 25,* 19-29.

Brody, J.A. (1982). Life expectancy and the health of the older person. *Journal of the American Geriatric Society, 30,* 681-683.

Brody, S.J., Poulshock, W., & Masciocchi, C. (1978). The family caring unit: A major consideration in the long-term support system. *Gerontologist, 18,* 556-561.

Burr, W.R. (1979). Role transitions: A reformulation of theory. *Journal of Marriage and the Family, 34,* 407-417.

Burr, W.R., Leigh, G.K., Day, R.D., & Constantine, J. (1979). Symbolic interaction and the family. In W. Burr, R. Hill, R.I. Nye, & I.L. Reiss, I.L. (Eds.), *Contemporary theories about the family,* Vol II.(pp. 47 & 72-111). New York: Raven Press.

Cantor, M.H. (1983). Strain among caregivers: A study of experience in the United States. *Gerontologist, 32,* 597-604.

Capitman, J. (1986). Community-based long-term care models, target groups, and impact on service use. *Gerontologist, 26,* 289-397.

Capitman, J., Haskins, B., & Bernstein, J. (1986). Case management approaches in coordinated community-oriented long-term care demonstrations. *Gerontologist, 26,* 398-404.

Cassel, F.(1976). The contribution of the social environment to host resistance. *American Journal of Epidemiology, 104* (2), 107-123.

Chappell, N. (1985). Social support and the receipt of home care services. *Gerontologist, 25,* 27-54.

Clark, N., & Rakowski, W. (1983). Family caregivers of older adults: Improving helping skills. *Gerontologist, 23,* 637-642.

Crossman, L., London, C., & Barry, C. (1981). Older women caring for disabled spouses: A model for supportive services. *Gerontologist, 21,* 464-470.

Doty, P. (1986). Family care of the elderly: The role of public policy. *Milbank Quarterly, 64* (1), 34-75.

Eggert, G., Granger, C., Morris, R., & Pendleton, S. (1977). Caring for the patient with long-term disability. *Geriatrics, 22,* (10) 102-114.

Feller, B.A. (1983). Need for care among the non institutionalized elderly. *Health: United States and Prevention Profile.* Md: USDHHS.

Fengler, A.P., & Goodrich, N. (1979). Wives of elderly disabled men: The hidden patients. *Gerontologist, 19* (2), 175-183.

Gilhooly, M. (1984). The impact of care-giving on care-givers: Factors associated with psychological well-being of people supporting a dementing relative in the community. *British Journal of Medical Psychology, 57,* 35-44.

Goldfarb, A.I.(1965). Psychodynamics and the three-generation family. In E. Shanas & G.F. Streib (Eds.). *Social structure and the family: Generational relations* (pp. 10-45). Englewood Cliffs, NJ: Prentice Hall.

Goode, W.J. (1960). A theory of role strain. *American Sociological Review, 25,* 483-496.

Grad, J. & Sainsbury, P. (1963). Mental illness and the family. *Lancet, 1,* 544-547.

Grad, J. & Sainsbury, P. (1968). The effects that patients have on their families in a community care and a control psychiatric service – a two year follow up. *British Journal of Psychiatry, 114,* 265-278.

Gurland, B., Copeland, J., Kuriansky, J., Kelleher, M., Sharpe, L., & Dean, L.L. (1983). *The mind and mood of aging.* New York: Haworth Press.

Guterman, S., & Dobson, A. (1986). Impact of the medicare prospective payment system for hospitals. *Health Care Financing Administration, 7* (3), 97-114.

Henry, J. (1982). The relation of social to biological processes in disease. *Social Science Medicine, 16,* 369-380.

Herz, M., Endicott, J., & Spitzer, R. (1976). Brief versus standard hospitalizations: The families. *American Journal of Psychiatry, 133,* 795-801.

Hoeing, J. & Hamilton, M. (1967). The burden on the household in extramural psychiatric service. In H. Freeman (Ed.). *New aspects of the mental health services.* (pp. 612-635). London: Pergamon Press.

Hooyman, N., Gonyea, J., & Montgomery, R. (1985). The impact of in-home services termination on family caregivers. *Gerontologist, 25,* 141-145.

Hooyman, N., & Lustbader, W. (1986). *Taking care: Supporting older people and their families.* New York: Free Press.

Horn, B.(Principal Investigator), (1986). *Elderly homecare project.* (Unpublished preliminary report). Funded by Fred Meyer Charitable Trust. Seattle, WA: University of Washington, School of Nursing, Community Health Care Systems.

Horowitz, A. (1985). Sons and daughters as caregivers to older parents: Differences in role performance and consequences. *Gerontologist, 25,* 612-617.

Johnson, C. & Catalano, D. (1983). A longitudinal study of family support to impaired elderly. *Gerontologist, 23* (6), 612-618.

Kahn, R. & Antonucci, T. (1980). Convoys over the life course; Attachment, roles, and social support. *Life Span Development and Behavior, 3,* 353-286.

Kohen, J. (1983). Old but not alone: Informal social supports among the elderly by marital status and sex. *Gerontologist, 23,* 57-63.

Liem, P, Chernoff, R., & Carter, W. (1986). Geriatric rehabilitation unit: Outcome evaluation. *Journal of Gerontology, 41,* 44-50.

Litwak, E. (1985). *Helping the elderly.* New York: Guilford Press.

McCubbin, H., Joy, C., Cauble, Comeau, J., Patterson, J., & Needle, R. (1980). Family stress and coping: A decade review. *Journal of Marriage and the Family, 42,* 885-868.

McKinley, J. (1981). Social network influences on morbid episodes and the career of help seeking. In L. Eisenberg & A. Kleinman (Eds.). *Culture illness and healing,* (pp. 77-104). Boston: D. Reidel Publishing Co.

Martin, D., Morycz, R., McDowell, J., Snustad, D., & Karpf, M. (1985). Community-based geriatric assessment. *Journal of American Geriatrics Society, 33* (9), 602-606.

Montgomery, R. (1986). Consultation conference with Elderly Homecare Project. University of Washington, School of Nursing.

Montgomery, R., Gonyea, J., & Hooyman, N. (1985). Caregiving and the experience of subjective and objective burden. *Family Relations, 34,* 19-26.

Montgomery, R., Stull, D., & Borgatta, E. (1985). Measurement and analysis of burden. *Research on Aging, 7* (1), 137-152.

National Center for Health Statistics (1984). *Vital Statistics of the United States: 1979 Volume II – Mortality, Part A.* MD: USDHHS.

Nydegger, S.N. (1983). Family ties of the aged in cross cultural perspective. *Gerontologist, 23* (1), 23-31.

Peszcnecker, B. & Zahlis, E. (1986). Establishing mutual-help groups for the family-member care givers: A new role for community health nurses. *Public Health Nursing, 3* (1), 29-37.

Platt, S., & Hirsch, S. (1981). The effects of brief hospitalization upon the psychiatric patient's household. *Acta Psychiatrica Scandinavaca, 64,* 199-216.

Poulshock, S., & Deimling, G. (1984). Families caring for elders in residence: Issues in measurement of burden. *Journal of Gerontology, 39,* 230-239.

Robinson, B. (1983). Validation of a caregiver strain index. *Journal of Gerontology, 38* 344-348.

Robinson, B. & Thurnher, M. (1979). Taking care of aged parents: A family cycle transition. *Gerontologist, 19* (6), 586-593.

Sanford, J.R. (1975). Tolerance of debility in elderly dependents by supporters at home: Its significance for hospital practice. *British Medical Journal, 3*, 471-473.

Scott, J. & Roberto, K. (1985). Use of informal and formal support networks by rural elderly poor. *Gerontologist, 25,* 624-630.

Seelbach, W.C. (1977). Gender differences in expectations for filial responsibility. *Gerontologist, 17,* 421-425.

Silliman, R., Fletcher, R., Earp, J., & Wagner, E. (1986). Families of elderly stroke patients. *Journal of the American Geriatrics Society, 34,* 643-648.

Soldo, B. & Myllyluoma, J. (1983). Caregivers who live with dependent elderly. *Gerontologist, 23* (6), 605-611.

Stoller, E. & Earl, L. (1983). Help with activities of everyday life: Sources of support for the noninstitutionalized elderly. *Gerontologist,23,* 64-70.

Streib, G. & Beck, R. (1980). Older families: A decade review. *Journal of Marriage and the Family, 42,* 937-957.

Taylor, M. (1985). The effect of DRGs on home health care. *Nursing Outlook, 33,* 288-291.

Terkelsen, K.G. (1980). Toward a theory of the family life cycle. In E.A. Carter & M. McGoldrick (Eds). *The family life cycle.* (pp. 21-53). New York: Gardner Press.

Thompson E. & Doll, W. (1982). The burden of families coping with the mentally ill. An invisible crises. *Family Relations, 31,* 379-388.

Townsend, A. & Poulshock, W. (1986). Intergenerational perspectives on impaired elders' support networks. *Journal of Gerontology, 41,* 101-109.

Troll, L. (1971). The family in later life: A decade review. *Journal of Marriage and the Family, 33,* 263-290.

U.S. Bureau of Census (October 1982). Decennial censuses of the population, 1900-1980 and Projections of the population of the United States: 1982-2050 (advanced report). *Current Population Reports*, Series P-25, No. 922.

Williams, F., Hill, J., Fairbank, M., & Knox, G. (1973). Appropriate placement of the chronically ill and aged. *Journal of the American Medical Association, 226,* 1332-1335.

Zarit, S.H. Reever, K.E., & Bach-Peterson, J. (1980). Relatives of the impaired elderly: Correlates of feelings of burden. *Gerontologist, 20,* 649-655.

Zung, W. (1974). The measurement of affects: Depression and anxiety. *Psychological Measurements in Psychopharmacology, 7,* 170-188.

APPENDIX A

CAREGIVER ASSESSMENT AND PLANNING GUIDE

I. IDENTIFYING INFORMATION

Date: _____

Name: _____

Age: _____   Sex: _____

Address: _____   Caregiver for: _____

Phone No.: _____   Relationship: _____

Living Arrangements: _____

Emergency Contact for Caregiver: _____

    Name: _____

    Address: _____

    Phone No.: _____

    Distance in miles from Caregiver: _____

II. ESSENTIAL QUESTIONS FOR FIRST VISIT

QUESTIONS	RESPONSE (Caregiver's Answer)	COMMENTS & PLANS (Health Provider's Observations and Plan of Care)
1. Do you have any health problems that prevent you from providing any of the care?		
2. Are you able to manage all the necessary care?		
3. Do you know how to get help from health care agencies?		
4. Are there any family or other sources of help you are using right now for help with your own health or that of the one you care for? LIST . . .		
5. Are you having financial difficulty in getting the help you need?		

III. PROBLEM IDENTIFICATION

A. DOES THE PERSON YOU CARE FOR OR NEED HELP WITH ANY OF THE FOLLOWING?

Problems Area	Do you have this problem?			If yes ask: how hard is it for you to deal with this problem?				Comments & Plans?
	No	OCC	Yes	Very Hard	Pretty Hard	Not too Hard	Easy	
	0	1	2	4	3	2	1	
1. Lifting?	0	1	2	4	3	2	1	
2. Urinary problems?	0	1	2	4	3	2	1	
3. Bowel problems?	0	1	2	4	3	2	1	
4. Need to be checked on at night?	0	1	2	4	3	2	1	
5. Management of disruptive or emotional problems?	0	1	2	4	3	2	1	
6. Poor hearing?	0	1	2	4	3	2	1	
7. Poor eye sight?	0	1	2	4	3	2	1	

171

Problems Area	No 0	OCC 1	Yes 2	Very Hard 4	Pretty Hard 3	Not too Hard 2	Easy 1	Comments & Plans?
8. Complicated medication schedule?	0	1	2	4	3	2	1	
9. Medical equipment?	0	1	2	4	3	2	1	
10. Other problems?								
a. _____	0	1	2	4	3	2	1	
b. _____	0	1	2	4	3	2	1	
c. _____	0	1	2	4	3	2	1	
d. _____	0	1	2	4	3	2	1	

III. PROBLEM IDENTIFICATION (cont. . .)

B. ARE YOU HAVING PROBLEMS WITH ANY OF THE FOLLOWING?

Problems Area	Do you have this problem?			If yes ask: how hard is it for you to deal with this problem?				Comments & Plans?
	NO	OCC	YES	Very Hard	Pretty Hard	Not too Hard	Easy	
	0	1	2	4	3	2	1	
1. Getting sleep?	0	1	2	4	3	2	1	
2. Health problems that are not being treated?	0	1	2	4	3	2	1	
3. Fatigue or weakness?	0	1	2	4	3	2	1	
4. Taking medications more frequently for nerves or sleep?	0	1	2	4	3	2	1	
5. Unintentional weightloss?	0	1	2	4	3	2	1	
6. Poor health?	0	1	2	4	3	2	1	

173

	NO	OCC	YES	Very Hard	Pretty Hard	Not too Hard	Easy
	0	1	2	4	3	2	1
7. Overwhelmed by situation?	0	1	2	4	3	2	1
8. Feeling not doing a good job of giving care?	0	1	2	4	3	2	1
9. Isolation from usual activities?	0	1	2	4	3	2	1
10. No time away from caregiving?	0	1	2	4	3	2	1
11. Unable to meet other responsibilities to family, friends or jobs?	0	1	2	4	3	2	1
12. Conflict with family over what care is needed for one you care for?	0	1	2	4	3	2	1

IV. MAJOR STRESSES, STRENGTHS, AND SUPPORT

QUESTIONS	RESPONSE (Caregiver's Answer)	COMMENTS & PLANS (Health Provider Observations and Plan of Care)
1. Have there been any major changes that you have had to deal with over the past year (moves, losses, family problems)?		
2. What have you found as sources of strength during these changes?		
3. What are you finding most difficult in giving care?		

QUESTIONS	RESPONSE (Caregiver's Answer)	COMMENTS & PLANS (Health Provider Observations and Plan of Care)
4. How have you been able to manage the difficulties?		
5. What are you finding most stressful about the caregiving situation?		
6. What helps you in relieving the stress?		
7. What people provide you with the most help and support with caregiving?		
8. What people besides the person you care for counts on you for help or support?		

V. PLAN OF CARE:

APPENDIX B

CAPG EVALUATION FORM

Please rate the Caregiver Assessment Guide on the following:
CIRCLE your rating.

	Poor (1)	Fair (2)	Good (3)	Very Good (4)	Excellent (5)
1. Clarity of the instructions for using the guide........	1	2	3	4	5
2. Clarity of questions to the caregiver..........	1	2	3	4	5
3. Format of Essential Questions sections for ease of use	1	2	3	4	5
4. Format of Problems Identification section for ease of use..............	1	2	3	4	5
5. Format of Major Stresses Strengths and Support section for ease of use.............	1	2	3	4	5
6. Overall helpfulness of guide in identifying ways to support the caregiver................	1	2	3	4	5

7. How long did it take you to fill out the assessment guide?

8. Any comments you would like to make concerning use of this guide with this client?

APPENDIX C

OVERALL EVALUATION FORM

After using the Caregiver Assessment Guide five times, use this form after all of the prior five have been completed. Use this one form to judge your overall impression of the form after having used it five times. CIRCLE your rating.

	Poor (1)	Fair (2)	Good (3)	Very Good (4)	Excellent (5)
1. Clarity of the instructions for using the guides.......	1	2	3	4	5
2. Clarity of questions to the caregiver..........	1	2	3	4	5
3. Format of Essential Questions sections for ease of use	1	2	3	4	5
4. Format of Problems Identification section for ease of use..............	1	2	3	4	5
5. Format of Major Stresses Strengths and Support section for ease of use..............	1	2	3	4	5
6. Overall helpfulness of guides in identifying ways to support the caregiver................	1	2	3	4	5

7. Is this information you already collect on other forms?_____

8. Did the ratings in the Problem Identification section help you prioritize problems?_____

9. What suggestions and comments would you have regarding the guide?

_____

_____

_____

_____

Please use the back of this form for further comments if you like.

APPENDIX D

INSTRUCTIONS FOR USE OF CAREGIVER ASSESSMENT AND PLANNING GUIDE

The attached Caregiver Assessment form is to be used for family members who must care for an ill elderly person. The purpose of the assessment is to ensure that the family caregiver is able to provide the needed care without jeopardizing his or her own health. It can provide the information needed for developing a plan of care with the caregiver. It is to be used as a screen to determine if a more in-depth evaluation is necessary. It can be used by either a social worker or a nurse.

There are five parts to the assessment guide:

    I.   Identifying Information
    II.   Problems in Providing Care
   III. Effect of Caregiving on a Caregiver's Life
   IV. Major Stresses, Strengths, and Supports
    V. Plan of Care

    I.   Identifying Information:
        Fill out as directed.

    II.   Problem in Providing Care:
        These questions have to do with the caregiver's ability to manage caregiving tasks. By requesting the caregiver to rate them, the clinician can determine which ones need to be given priority.

   III. Effect of Caregiving on Caregiver's Life:
        This section has to do with the caregiver's health, feelings about the situation, and social life and roles other than caregiving. If the caregiver says yes to a problem, then the level of difficulty is determined to help set priorities in planning.

IV. Major Stresses, Strengths, and Support:
This section is to help the health professional to discover the caregiver's most pressing problems and to assess strengths and resources already being used by the client.

V. Plan of Care:
The plan of care can refer to problems by the numbers listed in the preceding sections. Then the client and the clinician can decide together on a plan of care.

CAREGIVER ASSESSMENT AND PLANNING GUIDE

IDENTIFYING INFORMATION : CAREGIVER

Name: _____   Date: _____

CARE-RECIPIENT (CLIENT)

Address: _____

Phone No: _____   Client's Age: _____ Sex: _____

Age: _____ Sex: _____   Client's Name: _____

How long have you provided care? _____   Relationship of Client to Caregiver: _____

Marital Status: _____   Lives with Caregiver? Yes _____ No _____

Emergency contact for Caregiver: _____
                                    (Name)   (Phone No)

II. PROBLEMS IN PROVIDING CARE: Does the person you care for need help with any of the following?
If yes: Ask how hard is it for you to deal with this problem?

	No	Yes	Easy	Not too Hard	Pretty Hard	Very Hard	Comments
1. Getting up and down from a bed or chair?	1	2	1	2	3	4	
2. Toileting?	1	2	1	2	3	4	
3. Dressing?	1	2	1	2	3	4	
4. Bathing?	1	2	1	2	3	4	
5. Eating food?	1	2	1	2	3	4	
6. Walking?	1	2	1	2	3	4	
7. Needs to be checked on all night?	1	2	1	2	3	4	
8. Management of disruptive emotional problems?	1	2	1	2	3	4	
9. Poor hearing?	1	2	1	2	3	4	
10. Poor eyesight?	1	2	1	2	3	4	
11. Taking medications?	1	2	1	2	3	4	
12. Medical equipment?	1	2	1	2	3	4	
13. Other problems?							
A. _____	1	2		2	3	4	
B. _____	1	2		2	3	4	

III. EFFECT OF CAREGIVING ON CAREGIVER'S LIFE. Are you having problems with any of the following?
If yes ask: How hard is it for you to deal the this problem?

	No	Yes	Easy	Not too Hard	Pretty Hard	Very Hard	Comments
14. Getting sleep?	1	2	1	2	3	4	
15. Health problems that are not being treated?	1	2	1	2	3	4	
16. Fatigue or weakness?	1	2	1	2	3	4	
17. Taking medications more frequently for nerves or sleep?	1	2	1	2	3	4	
18. Unintentional weight loss?	1	2	1	2	3	4	
19. Poor health?	1	2	1	2	3	4	
20. Feeling overwhelmed by the situation?	1	2	1	2	3	4	
21. Feeling unable to give good care?	1	2	1	2	3	4	
22. Feeling isolated or alone?	1	2	1	2	3	4	
23. No time away from caregiving?	1	2	1	2	3	4	
24. Unable to meet other responsibilities to family, friends or job?	1	2	1	2	3	4	
25. Conflict with family over what care is being provided?	1	2	1	2	3	4	

IV. MAJOR STRESSES, STRENGTHS AND SUPPORT

26. What do you think is your main problem in providing care right now?

27. How are you able to handle the problem?

28. What is your biggest concern for yourself?

29. What are you able to do about it?

30. What do you see as your strengths in handling the problems?

31. What or who provides you with the most help or support?

32. What do you hope for, plan for as far as an outcome is concerned?

V. PLAN OF CARE

APPENDIX E

Resources for Family Caregivers and Home Health Agencies

<u>Family Caregiver Resources</u>

Mace, N., & Robins, P. (1981). <u>The 36-hour Day: A Family Guide to Caring for Persons with Alzheimer's Disease, Related Dementing Illnesses and Memory Loss in Later Life.</u> Baltimore: John Hopkins University.

Pacific Northwest Extension (1984). <u>Aging Parents: Helping When Health Fails.</u> Oregon State University Extension Service: PNW 246.

Pacific Northwest Extension (1985). <u>Families and Aging: A Guide to Legal Concerns.</u> Oregon State University Extension Service: Extension Circular 1221.

Silverstone, B., & Hyman, H.K. (1982). <u>You and Your Aging Parent.</u> New York: Pantheon.

<u>Home Health Agency Resources</u>

Applebaum, R.A., & Austin, C.D. <u>A Guide to the Evaluation of Long-term Care Case Management Programs.</u> Available through Institute on Aging JM-20 University of Washington, 3935 University Way NE, Seattle, WA (206) 543-8727

<u>Family Seminars for Care Giving: Helping Families Help</u> A Facilitators Guide and A Participants Handbook Available through Institute on Aging, University of Washington JM-20, Seattle, WA 98195

Hooyman, N., & Lustbader, W. (1986). <u>Taking Care: Supporting Older People and Their Families.</u> New York: Free Press.

Montgomery, R., & Prothero, J. (Eds.). <u>Developing Respite Services for the Elderly.</u> Available through University of Washington Press, P.O. Box C-50096, Seattle, WA 98145 (206) 543-4050.

O'Connor, K., & Prothero, J. (Eds.). <u>The Alzheimer's Caregiver: Strategies for Support.</u> Available through University of Washington, P.O. Box C-50096, Seattle, WA 98145

APPENDIX F

Contributors' Bibliographic Information

Patricia Archbold, RN, DNSc, FAAN
Consultant
Associate Professor, Family Nursing
Oregon Health Science University
Portland, Oregon 97201

Barbara Horn, RN Ph.D.
Principal Investigator
Professor, Community Health Care Systems SM-24
University of Washington
Seattle, Washington 98195

Rhonda Montgomery, Ph.D.
Consultant
Director of Institute of Gerontology
Wayne State University
Detriot, Michigan 48202

Barabara Stewart Ph.D.
Consultant
Professor
Office of Research Development and Utilization
School of Nursing
Oregon Health Science University
Portland, Oregon 97201

Martha Worcester RN MS Predoctoral student
Research Associate
School of Nursing SM-24
University of Washington
Seattle, Washington 98195

For Product Safety Concerns and Information please contact our EU
representative GPSR@taylorandfrancis.com Taylor & Francis Verlag GmbH,
Kaufingerstraße 24, 80331 München, Germany

Printed and bound by CPI Group (UK) Ltd, Croydon, CR0 4YY
01/05/2025
01858509-0001